4 Weeks to Healthy Digestion

A Harvard Doctor's Proven Plan for Reducing Symptoms of

Diarrhea • Constipation • Heartburn • and More

Norton J. Greenberger, M.D.
Clinical Professor of Medicine, Harvard Medical School
with Roanne Weisman

New York Chicago San Francisco Lisbon London Madrid Mexico City
Milan New Delhi San Juan Seoul Singapore Sydney Toronto

The *McGraw·Hill* Companies

Library of Congress Cataloging-in-Publication Data

Greenberger, Norton, J.
    4 weeks to healthy digestion : a harvard doctor's proven plan for reducing
symptoms of diarrhea, constipation, heartburn, and more / by Norton Greenberger
and Roanne Weisman.
        p.   cm.
    Includes index.
    ISBN-13: 978-0-07-154795-6 (alk. paper)
    ISBN-10:   0-07-154795-9 (alk. paper)
    1. Gastrointestinal system—Dieases—Popular works.   I. Weisman, Roanne,
1952–. II. Title.

RG806.G74 2009
616.3'306—dc22   2008038144

2 3 4 5 6 7 8 9 10 11 12 13 14 15 16 17 18 19 20 21 22 DOC/DOC 0 9

ISBN 978-0-07-154795-6
MHID   0-07-154795-9

Figures I.1, 2.1, 2.2, 3.1, 5.1, 6.1, and 8.1 by Scott Leighton; Figures 4.1 and 4.2 by
Michael Linkinhoker; Figure 7.1 by Christopher Bing

Additional nutritional analysis for select recipes on pages 152–217 provided by
Bethany Klos, RD, LDN

McGraw-Hill books are available at special quantity discounts to use as premiums and
sales promotions or for use in corporate training programs. To contact a representative,
please visit the Contact Us pages at www.mhprofessional.com.

This book is printed on acid-free paper.

Contents

Introduction

Some people have an "iron stomach" and can eat or drink anything without a problem. You probably know a few of these people! That exceptional group not withstanding, most of us do react to what we eat or drink. For some, indigestion happens only rarely, as a result of overindulging in the wrong kinds of food or drink choices, while for others—and you may be in this category—digestion problems happen much more often.

Living with a Sensitive Stomach

You are probably interested in this book because you have a sensitive stomach: a gastrointestinal (GI) system that reacts strongly to what you put into it. This is called *visceral hyperalgesia*, which simply means that you have chronic GI distress. Symptoms of your distress might include diarrhea, constipation, heartburn (also called gastroesophageal reflux disease, or GERD), dyspepsia (recurrent abdominal pain), bloating, or gas.

The problem with such chronic GI distress is that it's what is called a functional disorder, which means that there is nothing *structurally wrong* with your digestion system. There is also no disease present that can be "cured." You and your doctor may be frustrated because there is usually no one thing you can do—no pill to take, no operation to undergo—that will make the problem go away. So, how do you cope?

Living with a sensitive gut takes understanding, a positive attitude, and a commonsense approach to managing your temperamental digestion. The understanding and the commonsense approach will, I hope, come from this book. Your positive attitude may come from the fact that while your digestion problems are both real and difficult, they are not life threatening. Moreover, as you will see as you read further, they do not have to be a burden or interfere with your daily activities.

How to Use This Book

The focus of this book—as well as of the Four-Week Plan for Healthy Digestion—is first and foremost on healthy nutrition. As the saying goes, you are what you eat. I would expand that concept to digestion: your digestion depends on what and even *how* you eat. Every digestion problem discussed in this book is closely tied not only to everything that goes into your mouth—including foods, beverages, medications, vitamins, supplements, snacks, and even that after-dinner mint—but also to your method of eating. For example, do you "inhale" your food without taking the time to chew it fully? Do you eat in an atmosphere of stress? These habits are not conducive to digestive health. By contrast, calm, slow mealtimes and chewing every bite thoroughly both help to improve your digestion.

The key to a healthy, comfortable digestion is *mindfulness* about what you eat and how you eat, as well as close attention to your symptoms. To help you, I have included a Food and Symptom Log in Chapter 1 as a template for you to record this information. The log you maintain will give you an excellent point of reference to begin discussing the best digestion solutions with your doctor. Chapter 9, "Communicating with Your Doctor," offers suggestions on how to do this.

The first chapter describes the Four-Week Plan in general terms. Chapters on specific symptoms follow, and you can pick and choose the sections that apply to you. In those chapters, you will find more detailed guidance about using the Four-Week Plan, including which foods to avoid or include, as well as any specific lifestyle changes that apply. If you are a woman, Chapter 8, "For Women Only," will be of interest, since your gut reacts to your female hormones, as well as to your menstrual cycle and to menopause. Finally, for anyone who likes to cook, Part 2 has some delicious and digestion-friendly recipes, organized according to symptom.

About Me

In more than forty-five years of practicing, teaching, and writing about gastrointestinal medicine, I have seen thousands of patients with complaints just like the ones that you may be enduring: painful and uncomfortable digestive problems that interfere with daily life. In caring for these patients, I have come to two important realizations:

- Most people do not recognize the extent to which their dietary habits can cause recurrent gastrointestinal distress.
- Many doctors do not take the time to probe the diet and eating habits of their patients by taking a complete dietary history.

These two determinations are what prompted me to write this book—my first for the general public, although I have written or contributed to many textbooks and journal articles. I have written this book to help people understand how the gastrointestinal system works. When you have that understanding, it is often easy to adopt simple lifestyle and diet changes that will resolve, or at least alleviate, your digestion problems.

Before going any further, I'd like to introduce you to your digestive system! The following section may give you some surprising information about the complex and precisely coordinated group of organs packed into your abdomen. Read on to discover how the system is *supposed* to work. This will give you a better understanding of what happens when things go wrong—and how to regain proper digestive functioning.

▶Your Gastrointestinal System:
More than Digestion

Two glorious scoops of gourmet ice cream are waiting in a bowl in front of you. You pick up your spoon, anticipating the sweetness of that first cold, creamy taste.

This is hardly the time you want to be thinking about your gastrointestinal system, but indulge me for a moment, since that is what this book is about. You may be reading this book because you are having some problems with your digestion. The Four-Week Plan is designed to help you manage these problems, but before we launch into the plan, it is important to understand the gastrointestinal system and how it is supposed to work.

One way to think of your gastrointestinal system is as a twenty-five-foot-long "processing plant" that is compactly folded so that it fits into your abdomen. The largest part of this system is the *alimentary canal*, described in detail later. Everything that goes into your mouth, including food, beverages, medications, and any nutritional supplements, passes through this canal before it leaves your body. The GI system does far more than transport food, however. Before the food leaves your body, the system also breaks it down into molecules of substances that your body needs in order to live—proteins, carbohydrates, fats, vitamins, minerals, and water. It then delivers these vital sources of life and health directly into your bloodstream, which carries the nutrients to every cell, tissue, and organ. Connected to the alimentary canal are several "accessory" organs that produce digestive juices, enzymes, and acids that help break down the food. Whatever nutrients your body does not use for "fuel"—nourishment —are discarded as stool or urine.

What Is the Alimentary Canal?

The alimentary canal begins in the mouth and throat, through which food passes on its way to a muscular tube called the esophagus. The rhythmic contractions of the esophagus move food downward toward a muscular ring, called the esophageal sphincter, which opens at the appropriate time to allow food to pass through into the stomach. The stomach is connected to the small bowel (small intestine), which empties into the colon (large intestine). At the end of the journey is the rectum, which releases waste products as stool. Liquid waste is processed through the kidneys and bladder, passing out of the body through the urethra as urine. (See Figure I.1.)

Connected to various parts of the alimentary canal are three "accessory" organs: the liver, gallbladder, and pancreas, all of which

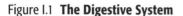

Figure I.1 **The Digestive System**

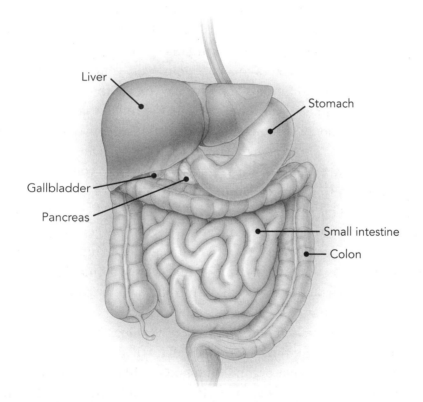

The drawing shows the lower part of the esophagus along with the stomach, liver, gallbladder, pancreas, small bowel or small intestine, and large bowel or colon. All of these organs play a leading role in healthy digestion.

interact with exquisite complexity and precision timing, beginning with that first bite of food. Working in concert, they release the precise amounts of digestive enzymes, acids, and juices needed at every stage of digestion, helping food and liquids move efficiently through the system.

A Symphony of Sustenance

Now, finally, let us return to that melting bowl of ice cream and watch how your gastrointestinal system responds to it. Each organ in the system has a part to play, at a particular time, almost as if it were a member of an orchestra being cued into action by an invisible conductor. In the GI system, the "conductors" of this "symphony of sustenance" are actually hormones—chemical messengers—released by the stomach and small intestine in the presence of food. These hormones trigger the timed production of digestive enzymes, acids, and juices in the organs of the GI system.

First, even before you take a bite, your eyes, your sense of smell, and even your imagination are preparing you for the treat to come: The salivary glands in your mouth begin to produce saliva in anticipation. (If you doubt the power of your mind to affect your digestion, try just *thinking* about chewing on a piece of fresh lemon, and notice the extra saliva in your mouth!) As you put food into your mouth, the saliva is ready to work, moistening the food to make it easier for the teeth to grind into smaller pieces for swallowing. This ice cream, of course, needs no chewing, but meat and vegetables certainly do, and as I point out in Chapters 1 and 5, sufficient chewing is important for healthy digestion. When the food reaches the stomach, enzymes, digestive juices, and acids break it into still smaller pieces, sending it down to the first part of the small bowel, which triggers the gallbladder to squeeze and contract, releasing juices and bile into the small bowel to break the food down still further.

The liver, the largest organ in the body, is like a factory, producing proteins and bile that are stored in the gallbladder until they are needed for digestion. The liver also stores iron, vitamins, and trace elements from the food you eat. One of the most important liver functions is to act as the body's "detoxifier," metabolizing all foods, beverages, and medicines to remove harmful elements before sending them back out into the body so that they can be effectively used and their by-products can be easily excreted. (Drinking too much alcohol can put a strain on the liver's detoxifying process and, if carried out over years, can cause it to enlarge, which can result in cirrhosis. This is a condition in which the liver becomes scarred and all of its functions are compromised.)

When food enters the small bowel, it also triggers the pancreas to release pancreatic enzymes that help digest proteins, fats, and carbohydrates. The pancreas also releases insulin, which is important in metabolizing sugars. (A deficiency of insulin results in diabetes. Chapter 7 features the specific digestion problems of people with diabetes.) Together, the bile salts from the gallbladder and the pancreatic juices break down these food substances into molecules that can be absorbed across the lining of the small bowel into the bloodstream and transported throughout the body. After this digestion has taken place, the breakdown products stop the pancreas and gallbladder from producing their enzymes and acids, again with perfect timing.

Any food products that are not absorbed through the lining of the small bowel continue into the colon (large intestine), a wider tube that is shorter than the small bowel. In the colon, bacteria work to digest any remaining food. The upper part of the colon also absorbs remaining fluids and bile salts. Anything left over is waste that the body does not need, so muscle contractions push it into the rectum, where it is stored until it is ready to be released through the anus as a bowel movement.

To return to your ice cream: When it enters the first part of the small bowel, it triggers the release of bile and pancreatic juices. When the digestion of the ice cream is complete, the upper bowel releases chemicals that "turn off" the pancreas and the gallbladder. The digested sugars and fats from the ice cream are then ready to be absorbed. This summary illustrates the exquisite regulation of something as simple as eating ice cream.

In all, it takes about six to twelve hours for that ice cream to make its way through the entire gastrointestinal system. A heavier meal, especially if it contains fat, will slow the stomach down and extend the digestive process. As you read through the GI "problem" chapters that follow, it may be useful to refer back to this section for a better understanding of which processes are being interfered with and how you can use the Four-Week Plan to restore a healthy gut!

Healthy Digestion

I hope that this understanding of your gastrointestinal system has inspired you to begin the Four-Week Plan to reduce uncomfortable symptoms and reclaim your digestive health. If you are ready, start with Chapter 1 to learn how the Four-Week Plan can help you. Here's to your healthy digestion!

PART 1

· ·

What You Need to Know About Healthy Digestion

Introducing the Four-Week Plan for Healthy Digestion

The Four-Week Plan for Healthy Digestion that I present in this book is designed to set you on a course that will not only relieve your symptoms now but also stay with you as permanent lifestyle changes to prevent digestion problems in the future. Even if you go "off the wagon" and your symptoms recur, you can always use the plan to realign your lifestyle and eating habits once again, for a lifetime of trouble-free digestion. In this chapter, I outline the plan for you, to give you an idea of what happens during each week. Do not make any changes yet in response to what you read; just begin to think about your own digestion problems. Then, you can go directly to the chapter (or chapters) in which your problems are addressed specifically and put the plan into action. When you are ready, the delicious recipes in Part 2 will help you enjoy trouble-free eating!

The First Week: Start Your Food and Symptom Log

A key part of the Plan for Healthy Digestion is awareness. As you become more conscious of what you eat and drink and of the effects of certain foods and beverages on your body, you begin to acquire the power of knowledge. With knowledge comes the power to change. During the first week, you will begin to collect vital information about your diet and your body that will help you and your doctor discover the best ways to control your symptoms. Your main tool will be your Food and Symptom Log, which is simply a written record of everything you eat and drink, as well as of your gastrointestinal symptoms. Sample log pages are also included in this chapter, and later, I will show you how to collect this information.

This week, your first mission is to discover and record. Think of yourself as a detective collecting data. This is your "baseline" or "run-in" period. It forms the beginning of a fact-finding system that you will learn about in more detail later on. Your main task this week is to begin your log. You may be surprised at what it will reveal to you about your food choices! During the first week, begin to record everything that goes into your mouth—including such "incidentals" as candy, gum, and mints. At the same time, record all of your abdominal symptoms. Remember to enter everything you are drinking and how much of each, including tea, coffee, soda, juice, and water. Using the format provided in this chapter will make it easier for you to keep track of what you are eating and drinking and the digestive problems you are having. Depending on your preference you can either photocopy the blank log or use it as a model for your own log.

Being inclusive is essential because many common foods and liquids can cause abdominal discomfort and digestion problems. (In later chapters, you will learn which symptoms are linked to each.) Just a few examples of these well-known troublemakers:

- Orange juice
- Tomato juice
- Red wine
- Vinegar-based salad dressings
- Pancake syrup

- Honey
- All so-called sugarless foods—such as sugarless gum and mints (a prime offender) and apple juice

During this first week, *do not change the way you eat or what you eat and drink*, but observe and record everything carefully, along with the timing and severity of digestive problems. This undertaking will give you a baseline picture of the relationship between what you eat and how you feel. The sample log in this chapter illustrates what you might record during a typical four-week period.

Your 1–5 Intensity Scale

As part of your discovery process, you will use a scale of 1 through 5 to record the intensity of your symptoms. Both a template and sample log pages are included here.

As you can see, the "Symptom" column allows you to record whether a symptom is present and how severe it is. If no symptoms occur, leave blank.

1 = no symptoms
2 = minimal symptoms—you are aware of them, but they are not causing a major problem
3 = moderate symptoms, beginning to interfere with your life
4 = moderately severe symptoms, causing you to change your plans to accommodate them
5 = most severe symptoms, virtually incapacitating you

Duration of Symptoms

1 = less than 1 hour
2 = 1 hour
3 = 2 hours
4 = 3 hours
5 = greater than 3 hours

HOW TO FILL OUT YOUR FOOD AND SYMPTOM LOG

To help you get started on completing your Food and Symptom Log, I have prepared a simplified "sample" log, based on the experience of one of my patients. He is a sixty-four-year-old man who was having chronic diarrhea, but only at nighttime. The diarrhea was so severe that it woke him up at night, and occasionally, he would not make it to the bathroom in time. Curiously, the problem was most severe on Tuesdays and Thursdays. Look at Week 1 of the log to see what he wrote.

When we went over his log together, I noticed that he tended to eat a much larger quantity of food in the evening (this is typical of most people as dinner is often the biggest meal of the day), followed by fruit for dessert, which he loved. While ordinarily during the second week we do not usually recommend changes, I was impressed with his fruit, candy, and snack intake, and I opted to accelerate the process and suggest changes during the second week. So, to begin, I asked him to try to cut out all fresh fruit, candy, and other snacks, as you can see by looking at Week 2 of his log. The next week, his diarrhea was better, but he was still having the problem on Tuesday and Thursday nights. More detective work was needed! I suspected that he was leaving something out of his log. Sure enough, he was. He was attending a regular Alcoholics Anonymous group meeting on Tuesday and Thursday evenings, after dinner, at which he usually ate several cookies and drank fruit juices. The combination of cookies and fruit juices, with their load of simple sugars such as fructose, could well be contributing to his nighttime diarrhea on those two nights. Look at Week 2 of the sample log to see what he *should* have entered for Tuesdays and Thursdays.

For week three, I asked him to not to eat cookies and drink juice during the meetings. He decided, on his own, to substitute dietetic ice cream, which he recorded in his log. Look at Week 3 of his log to see this new information.

When we spoke at the end of that week, he told me he had followed my advice but was still having diarrhea on Tuesday and Thursday nights. The so-called sugarless ice cream that he was eating actually contains large amounts of sorbitol, which can cause diarrhea in otherwise healthy people.

"I'm sorry to have to ask you to do this," I said to him, "but during week four, I would like you to eat nothing at all during these meetings." He agreed to do so and reported back to me that the diarrhea was now gone. You can see that he recorded no symptoms during Week 4 of his log. After another two weeks with no symptoms, we worked together to find something that he *could* eat during these meetings. In addition to having one eight-ounce glass of water, he asked the organizers if he could bring some crackers and cheese, which he snacked on and also offered to the others at the meeting. This went so well that now crackers and cheese are part of the standard fare for these meetings. "I guess I have started a trend," he said, "and this works for me!"

The lesson here is: Do not leave *anything* out of your Food and Symptom Log, even if you think it is not important!

Over-the-Counter and Prescription Medications

Don't fail to record any medications that you are taking. Some *over-the-counter medicines* that you take regularly may actually be causing digestion problems such as nausea, abdominal discomfort, and constipation. These include the following:

- Aspirin
- Nonsteroidal drugs (Advil, ibuprofen, naproxen)
- Iron tablets
- Niacin (a vitamin)
- Antihistamines (can slow the stomach down)

SAMPLE FOOD AND SYMPTOM LOG†

WEEK 1

Day	Symptom* (Intensity: 1–5)**	Time of Day	Duration	Foods Eaten That Day
1 Sunday	Diarrhea 3	Night	30 min	Breakfast: bagel and cream cheese; Lunch: turkey sandwich, fruit; Snack: potato chips; Dinner: fish, potatoes, salad, fruit
2 Monday	Diarrhea 3	Night	30 min	Breakfast: bagel and cream cheese; Lunch: soup, fruit; Snack: trail mix; Dinner: chicken, potatoes, salad, fruit
3 Tuesday	Diarrhea 5	Night	2 hours	Breakfast: bagel and cream cheese; Lunch: turkey sandwich; Snack: candy bar; Dinner: fish, potatoes, salad, fruit
4 Wednesday	Diarrhea 3	Night	30 min	Breakfast: bagel and cream cheese; Lunch: turkey sandwich, fruit; Snack: potato chips; Dinner: chicken, potatoes, salad, fruit
5 Thursday	Diarrhea 5	Night	2 hours	Breakfast: bagel and cream cheese; Lunch: soup, fruit; Snack: potato chips; Dinner: seafood, potatoes, salad, fruit
6 Friday	Diarrhea 3	Night	30 min	Breakfast: bagel and cream cheese; Lunch: ham sandwich, fruit; Snack: trail mix; Dinner: cod, potatoes, salad, fruit

Day	Symptom* (Intensity: 1–5)**	Time of Day	Duration	Foods Eaten That Day
7 Saturday	Diarrhea 3	Night	30 min	Breakfast: bagel and cream cheese; Lunch: soup, fruit; Snack: candy bar; Dinner: chicken, potatoes, salad, fruit

WEEK 2

Day	Symptom* (Intensity: 1–5)**	Time of Day	Duration	Foods Eaten That Day
1 Sunday				Breakfast: bagel and cream cheese; Lunch: turkey sandwich; Snack: potato chips; Dinner: fish, potatoes, salad
2 Monday				Breakfast: bagel and cream cheese; Lunch: soup; Snack: trail mix; Dinner: chicken, potatoes, salad
3 Tuesday	Diarrhea 4	Night	1 hour	Breakfast: bagel and cream cheese; Lunch: turkey sandwich; Snack: crackers; Dinner: fish, potatoes, salad; Meeting: 4–6 cookies, 2 glasses apple juice
4 Wednesday				Breakfast: bagel and cream cheese; Lunch: turkey sandwich; Snack: potato chips; Dinner: chicken, potatoes, salad

(continued)

WEEK 2 *(continued)*

Day	Symptom* (Intensity: 1–5)**	Time of Day	Duration	Foods Eaten That Day
5 Thursday	Diarrhea 5	Night	2 hours	Breakfast: bagel and cream cheese; Lunch: soup, fruit; Snack: potato chips; Dinner: seafood, potatoes, salad, fruit Meeting: 4–6 cookies, 2 glasses apple juice
6 Friday	Diarrhea 3	Night	1 hour	Breakfast: bagel and cream cheese; Lunch: ham sandwich, fruit; Snack: trail mix; Dinner: cod, potatoes, salad
7 Saturday	Diarrhea 3	Night	30 min	Breakfast: bagel and cream cheese; Lunch: soup, fruit; Snack: candy bar; Dinner: chicken, potatoes, salad

WEEK 3

Day	Symptom* (Intensity: 1–5)**	Time of Day	Duration	Foods Eaten That Day
1 Sunday				Breakfast: bagel and cream cheese; Lunch: turkey sandwich; Snack: potato chips; Dinner: fish, potatoes, salad
2 Monday				Breakfast: bagel and cream cheese; Lunch: soup; Snack: trail mix; Dinner: chicken, potatoes, salad

Day				Food
3 Tuesday	Diarrhea 4	Night	1 hour	Breakfast: bagel and cream cheese; Lunch: turkey sandwich; Snack: peanut butter crackers; Dinner: fish, potatoes, salad; Meeting: 2 bowls of dietetic ice cream
4 Wednesday				Breakfast: bagel and cream cheese; Lunch: turkey sandwich; Snack: potato chips; Dinner: chicken, potatoes, salad
5 Thursday	Diarrhea 4	Night	1 hour	Breakfast: bagel and cream cheese; Lunch: turkey sandwich; Snack: corn chips; Dinner: fish, potatoes, salad, fruit; Meeting: 2 bowls of dietetic ice cream
6 Friday				Breakfast: bagel and cream cheese; Lunch: ham sandwich; Snack: trail mix; Dinner: cod, potatoes, salad
7 Saturday				Breakfast: bagel and cream cheese; Lunch: lasagna; Snack: peanut butter crackers; Dinner: chicken, potatoes, salad

(continued)

WEEK 4

Day	Symptom* (Intensity: 1–5)**	Time of Day	Duration	Foods Eaten That Day
1 Sunday				Breakfast: bagel and cream cheese; Lunch: turkey sandwich; Snack: potato chips; Dinner: fish, potatoes, salad
2 Monday				Breakfast: bagel and cream cheese; Lunch: soup, fruit; Snack: trail mix; Dinner: chicken, potatoes, salad
3 Tuesday				Breakfast: bagel and cream cheese; Lunch: turkey sandwich; Snack: peanut butter crackers; Dinner: fish, potatoes, salad
4 Wednesday				Breakfast: bagel and cream cheese; Lunch: turkey sandwich; Snack: potato chips; Dinner: chicken, potatoes, salad
5 Thursday				Breakfast: bagel and cream cheese; Lunch: turkey sandwich; Snack: corn chips; Dinner: fish, potatoes, salad
6 Friday				Breakfast: bagel and cream cheese; Lunch: ham sandwich; Snack: trail mix; Dinner: cod, potatoes, salad
7 Saturday				Breakfast: bagel and cream cheese; Lunch: lasagna; Snack: peanut butter crackers; Dinner: chicken, potatoes, salad

FOOD AND SYMPTOM LOG†
WEEK 1

Day	Symptom* (Intensity: 1–5)**	Time of Day	Duration	Foods Eaten That Day
1				
2				
3				
4				
5				
6				
7				

(continued)

WEEK 2

Day	Symptom* (Intensity: 1–5)**	Time of Day	Duration	Foods Eaten That Day
1				
2				
3				
4				
5				
6				
7				

WEEK 3

Day	Symptom* (Intensity: 1–5)**	Time of Day	Duration	Foods Eaten That Day
1				
2				
3				
4				
5				
6				
7				

(continued)

WEEK 4

Day	Symptom* (Intensity: 1–5)**	Time of Day	Duration	Foods Eaten That Day
1				
2				
3				
4				
5				
6				
7				

†If no symptoms occur on a particular day, leave blank.

*Symptom: Abdominal Pain (location);   Heartburn;   Dyspepsia;   Diarrhea;   Constipation;   Gas/Bloating

**Intensity: 1 = No symptoms;   2 = Minimal symptoms;   3 = Moderate symptoms;   4 = Moderately severe symptoms;   5 = Most severe symptoms

In addition to these, the following common *prescription medicines* can cause similar problems with your digestion:

- Antibiotics (including penicillin, amoxicillin, flagyl, erythromycin, cephalosporins, and Z pack—azithromycin
- High blood pressure medicines (many types)
- Antihistamines
- Colchicine (a gout medicine)
- Steroids
- Estrogens (depends in part on dose)

More detailed lists of problem medications appear in the symptom-specific chapters that follow. For this first week, it is enough just to keep track of everything you are taking. Again, *don't make any changes yet*. Just observe and record.

The Second Week: Change Your Eating Habits

You are off to a promising start! By now, you should be comfortable with your Food and Symptom Log and are probably wondering what happens next. This is the week to take a look at some of your lifestyle and eating habits. This is important because the way you eat, not just what you eat, affects both your digestion and how you feel.

So, during this second week, as you continue filling out your log, we are going to add a few activities. It is not time yet to make any changes in your diet itself, however. At the beginning of this week, take a moment to look back over the week you have just recorded. What do you notice? Do certain foods tend to trigger certain symptoms? At what time of day do your symptoms usually occur? You might begin to notice a pattern, and this noticing—what we call *mindfulness*—is going to be the ticket to your digestion relief. We will explore this aspect further later on, but for now, continue to gather information about your own body and its reactions to food.

This week, in addition to recording information, I am going to ask you to change your eating *behavior*—but we are not going to start eliminating food yet. That will happen during week three.

The Benefits of Portion Control

Eating too much is a major cause of digestive problems. But what is too much? What is a normal-size meal? How large should your plate of food be? There is no precise answer to these questions, but chances are you would have an easier time with digestion if you made your portion sizes and meals smaller. This is not easy to do! Over the past few decades, the sizes of our meals (also called portion sizes) have increased dramatically. Thanks to advertising, "supersizing," "all-you-can-eat" buffets, and so-called value meals (which are actually of negative value), we have become accustomed to eating large quantities of food. So, this week, I'd like you to cut down on your meal and portion sizes. How to do this? Here are some tips:

■ **Cut your normal food portions.** If you're hungry, add more vegetables.

■ **Use smaller plates, and put less on the plate.** Studies have shown that people will eat whatever is put in front of them. (That's probably because we were all trained to "clean our plates.")

■ **No seconds!** Don't go back for more food.

■ **Don't eat until you are "stuffed."** Learn to stop eating when you are no longer hungry. This is key. Train yourself to recognize your hunger level by asking yourself if you are hungry every few minutes while you are eating. Stop eating if you are no longer hungry. Often you will stop being hungry before you are "full" or "stuffed," and if you keep eating after this point, it could give you digestion problems.

Slowing Down

Eating too quickly is also an important cause of digestive issues. To avoid the tendency to "inhale" your food, strive to stretch mealtimes out to at least twenty minutes. Swallowing everything down in a few gulps and a few minutes is bad for your digestion. So is gobbling your breakfast in the car on the way to work. Rather, I'd like you to practice swallowing at least sixty times for each meal. Put your knife and fork down periodically and take a break; have an interesting conversation with your meal partners, or just relax for a moment or two before going on. Mealtimes should be relaxing, not food marathons! Another key to eating more slowly is to cut a piece of food, put down your knife, eat that piece, and then cut the next piece. Cutting all of your food into bite-size pieces before you begin eating encourages "inhaling" your food. Enjoy each bite, and chew it thoroughly.

Eating with Others

Families that eat dinner in shifts or on the run are at risk not only for indigestion but also for behavior problems among their children, according to research from the Columbia University Center on Addiction and Substance Abuse. Kids in families that have sit-down dinners together are far less likely to smoke, drink, and take drugs than kids whose families have more haphazard lifestyles. Regular family mealtimes also result in better grades and nutritional habits among children.

To keep mealtimes calm and relaxed, try to focus on topics that are interesting but that don't make you clench your stomach in anger! If you live alone, schedule some leisurely mealtimes with friends, colleagues, or family members.

Fantastic (and Not-So-Fantastic) Fluids

Sipping water with your meals is a good idea. Water reduces the caloric density of your food and dilutes material entering your bowel, for easier digestion.

While water is desirable, skip the sodas and some juices. Colas, for example, have forty grams of sugar and about 160 calories in sixteen ounces, none of which will help either your digestion or your waistline. Diet colas are usually not a problem, because they contain very small amounts of aspartame (Equal) or sucralose (Splenda). Both tomato juice and orange juice are acidic, meaning they might increase heartburn. If you have a tendency toward this problem, avoid them, not only with meals but also in general.

Other liquid digestion culprits include alcohol, caffeinated tea and coffee, and milk, all of which can worsen dyspepsia and acid reflux (also called heartburn or gastroesophageal reflux disease).

▶The Third Week: Eliminate Problem Foods

This week marks the beginning of what may become a significant change in your eating habits, because this is the week you will begin to eliminate problem-causing foods. As a first step, review your Food and Symptom Log once again, but this time, make a list of the foods and supplements or vitamins that are associated with your symptoms. This week, begin to sharply decrease your intake of those foods or, if you can, completely eliminate them from your diet. *Do not stop taking any medication without consulting your doctor.*

Your Food Profile

Continue your Food and Symptom Log and the new eating habits that you began last week—eating slowly; chewing thoroughly; using portion control; and replacing soda, juices, caffeinated beverages, alcohol, and milk with water. Carefully make note of any changes in your symptoms as a result of these changes in your diet. More than likely, you will notice some improvement. Each person reacts individually to food, and the goal of this program is to help you find your own personal food "profile."

Common Foods to Eliminate

The following are samples of some of the most common problem foods that you might be eliminating during week three, along with their associated conditions. These lists are just for informational purposes now. In the chapters that follow, I will give you a more detailed list of common digestion culprits for each condition.

Diarrhea

- Fruits, especially peaches, pears, cherries, and apples
- Fruit juices, especially apple and orange juice
- Beans and other high-fiber foods
- Coffee
- Dairy products such as milk, ice cream, and cheese, especially if you are lactose intolerant
- "Sugar-free" gum and snacks that contain sorbitol or sugar alcohols

Constipation

- Low-fiber foods, such as fast foods and prepared foods
- Simple carbohydrates, such as white rice, white bread, and pasta
- Eggs
- Meats

Dyspepsia and Heartburn
(Gastroesophageal Reflux Disease)

- Beverages: colas, coffee, caffeinated tea, acidic juices such as orange and tomato, milk and other dairy products, alcohol
- Spicy sauces
- Beans
- Fatty foods
- Fried foods
- Peppers
- Radishes

Bloating and Gas

- Beverages: apple juice, orange juice, milk, carbonated drinks, wine
- Brassica vegetables: asparagus, broccoli, brussels sprouts, cabbage, cauliflower
- Foods rich in fructose and sorbitol: "sugar-free" items, pancake and waffle syrup, apples, cherries, peaches, pears

■ Beans
■ Turnips
■ Corn
■ Cucumbers
■ Grapes and raisins
■ Nuts
■ Oats and other high-fiber foods
■ Onions

▶The Fourth Week: Charting Your New Course

By this time, you should be enjoying calm, slow mealtimes with a refined awareness of what you are eating and drinking. You will also probably be feeling better, having reduced or eliminated the foods that are causing you problems. During this fourth week, you will refine your new eating plan.

Begin by reintroducing—one at a time—the foods that you eliminated last week. Carefully record in your log what you are eating and any associated symptoms. This will sharpen your awareness of the most problematic foods for you. It doesn't mean you have to cut them out completely, but at least you can make a conscious decision of what to eat and when to eat it, knowing the likely effects. This is also a good time to discuss your Food and Symptom Log with your doctor, nurse-practitioner, or dietitian, in order to get suggestions of foods that are beneficial for your particular symptoms. (Please see Chapter 9 for more information on working with your doctor to alleviate digestion problems.) Most of my patients, at this point, are motivated to work with me to permanently change their eating habits in order to stay feeling well!

The Experimental Period

The refining period in the fourth week is essential to making sure you have pinpointed your food culprit. The first two weeks—

your fact-finding weeks—form a baseline or run-in period for our digestion-improvement plan. During the third week, you use the information recorded in your log and begin eliminating or reducing problematic foods and recording the results. If things improve, you reintroduce the food or drink during week four.

The system we are using can be characterized as "ABAB." During the first "A" period (the first two weeks), you simply record and observe. During the first "B" period (the third week), you eliminate a troublesome food or drink and watch to see if it makes a difference. During the fourth week (a second "A" period), if things improve, you reintroduce that food or drink and watch what happens. If nothing happens, that food or drink is not causing you digestion problems. If, on the other hand, you notice problems again, you go to the second "B" period and eliminate it once more. If your digestion gets better without that food or drink, you can put it on the list of your "digestion culprits."

You can use this ABAB structure repeatedly if you want to test one food at a time. If you have several foods or drinks to test, this fourth "week" may stretch out a bit longer than an actual week. That is fine. It is better to keenly observe and accurately identify your problem foods than to miss them, even if this takes a bit more time. This system is designed to be flexible, so modify it if necessary to meet *your* needs.

If you want to test multiple foods at the same time, you can use a slightly different structure, "ABCD." Here, you still use "A" as your baseline period and "B" to eliminate the most troublesome food or drink and record the results. The difference comes in period "C," when you eliminate a group of other foods and/or drinks that you suspect are also causing trouble, and see what happens. Then during "D," you reintroduce one food or drink at a time and record the results. While this coming-and-going might sound confusing, your log will help you keep track of what you are doing. In the specific symptom chapters, I will walk you through the process with foods that are related to each symptom.

Tips for Reintroducing Foods and Beverages into Your Diet

If you use the ABAB method to test different kinds of foods and beverages, it is best to reintroduce each type of food one at a time, for a day or so, and monitor your reaction. If there is no reaction, you can assume—at least for the time being—that this food is not one of your digestion culprits. If, instead, you have one of the symptoms described earlier, you can probably assume that this food or drink should be off your dietary "repertoire." If you do choose to indulge—say, at a party or special occasion—at least do so mindfully, and know that it might take you a day or two to recover. Only you can decide if this outcome is worth it!

If you use the ABCD method because you have concluded that there is one class of foods—say, dairy products—that is causing you the most problems, you might try to reintroduce several dairy products at once, to see what happens. The obvious problem with this approach is that you might miss a specific food item that works better for you. Some people, for example, can digest yogurt more easily than milk.

Adding Beneficial Foods

In addition to retesting potential problem foods, you can do something positive for your digestion during this fourth week by adding in new foods that may help your particular symptom. This step is part of charting your course to healthier digestion and nutrition. By increasing your repertoire of beneficial foods and improving your eating habits, while reducing or eliminating harmful foods, you are creating new eating patterns that will help you avoid digestion problems for your whole life. In each symptom chapter, I will direct you to foods that may help your condition, but you should always discuss this action first with your doctor.

Getting Down to Details

Now that you are familiar with the Four-Week Plan for Healthy Digestion, it is time to explore your own symptoms in more depth. The remaining chapters give you detailed instructions for personalizing the Four-Week Plan for the digestion symptoms that are causing you problems. They also include which foods and beverages to avoid, strategies for relieving your symptoms, and tips to create your own plan for healthy digestion and nutrition. The second part of the book contains recipes that are organized by symptom, to help you keep your healthy digestion long after you have completed the Four-Week Plan.

Chapter 2

Diarrhea

I f you suffer from chronic diarrhea, you know that it can be extremely disruptive. The endless trips to the bathroom, the cramps and bloating, and the general discomfort can get in the way of life. And if the condition itself is not trouble enough, you are constantly bombarded by potential solutions. The pharmacy aisles are lined with medications that promise relief, but these products don't always provide the results you need. The good news is that you *can* banish many of your diarrhea woes through some simple diet and lifestyle changes.

You've already learned about the Four-Week Plan, so now it's time to get specific and create your own personalized version for diarrhea. In this chapter, I'll provide you with some basic information about the causes and symptoms of diarrhea, along with the tools to analyze and work with your own condition, in consultation with your doctor. After reading this chapter, you will be ready and able to create a focused, individualized path to improved digestive health, with fewer bathroom breaks!

What Is Diarrhea?

Simply put, diarrhea is way too much of a good thing. Your body is supposed to process food, liquid, and everything else that you eat, and that function includes the production of a certain amount of stool. Sometimes, the delicate balance of the digestive system is thrown off, resulting in loose, uncomfortable stools that interrupt your day far too often. This leaves you feeling chained to the bathroom and often dehydrated as well. Diarrhea is considered chronic if it has persisted for at least two months.

You may not realize that every day, your digestive system (see Figure 2.1), particularly your small and large bowels (intestines), must process nearly nine quarts of fluid! Of course, that does not all come from the water, coffee, tea, juice, or other beverages that you drink, which typically account for only about two quarts of this total. Your body actually produces the rest of this fluid, in the form of saliva (one quart), digestive juices from the stomach and pancreas (about three quarts), bile from the gallbladder (one and a half quarts), and an additional one to two quarts of fluids produced in the intestines to aid in digestion. Your small and large bowels are responsible for helping your body absorb up to 99 percent of this fluid, with the result that a normal bowel movement—the waste products that your body eliminates from the food that you eat— usually contains only about one-fifth of a quart of water.

Normally, your bowels can efficiently handle both the fluids that you drink and those your body produces. Problems arise, however, when viruses, bacteria, certain foods, sweeteners, or disease irritate or alter the lining of the small or large bowel, preventing the absorption of this fluid.

▶Causes of Diarrhea

Before we get to diarrhea food culprits—some of which may surprise you—let's look at some common conditions that cause diarrhea.

Too Much Fluid
Drinking excessive amounts of the wrong kinds of fluid—more than two gallons a day of colas, juices, or teas—especially if this

is combined with poorly digested foods, can cause fluid overload, overwhelming your body's absorption capacity. (See Figure 2.1.) This disruption in the delicate fluid balance of your digestive system brings on diarrhea.

Figure 2.1 **Daily Fluid Digestion**

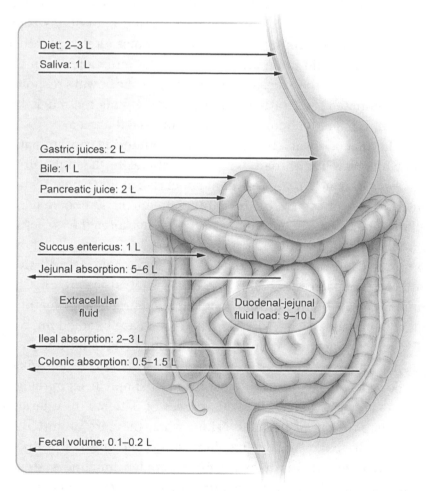

Diet: 2–3 L
Saliva: 1 L
Gastric juices: 2 L
Bile: 1 L
Pancreatic juice: 2 L
Succus entericus: 1 L
Jejunal absorption: 5–6 L
Extracellular fluid
Duodenal-jejunal fluid load: 9–10 L
Ileal absorption: 2–3 L
Colonic absorption: 0.5–1.5 L
Fecal volume: 0.1–0.2 L

Your digestive system processes several quarts of fluid a day. Here is where that fluid comes from, as expressed in liters (L). A quart is equivalent to 0.95 liters. Most of the fluid is absorbed, about one quart per day is eliminated in the urine, and up to half a pound of what is left is eliminated as stool. If the amount of fluids overwhelms your body's absorption or elimination capacity, diarrhea can occur.

Viral and Bacterial Gastroenteritis

Both bacteria and viruses can cause infections in your intestines, which irritate the lining of the bowel, resulting in inflammation, abdominal cramps, and diarrhea. Bacterial infections come from eating foods that are either handled improperly (such as by workers who don't wash their hands), improperly cooked (temperatures that are too low to kill bacteria), or contaminated by improper storage, allowing bacteria to grow. Viruses are transmitted from person-to-person contact. In response to either kind of gastroenteritis infection, the lining of the bowel becomes altered and then produces more fluid in an attempt to get the infection out of the body. In this case, the excess fluid is caused by the bowel's response to contaminated food, rather than by your drinking too much, but the result is similar: abdominal discomfort and diarrhea.

While you may be at a higher risk of encountering contaminated food while traveling abroad (which contributes to the high rate of "traveler's diarrhea"), you're still at some risk at your local restaurant, at home, or even in the hospital. Salmonella, E. coli, and Shigella are bacteria in contaminated foods that alter the structure of your intestinal lining and cause diarrhea. Salmonella shows up in raw or incompletely cooked poultry and eggs, as well as in spoiled or nonpasteurized dairy products, such as ice cream. Contaminated, raw, or incompletely cooked hamburger can sometimes have E. coli, and Shigella occurs when foods are handled improperly during production or during preparation in a restaurant.

A particularly deadly bacterium called *Clostridiuim difficile* may not come from any of these sources. It simply lives in the gut of many people. In fact, 20 to 40 percent of patients in American hospitals either have this bacterium when they are admitted or acquire it by exposure during their stay—but only half experience symptoms; this is because most people's immune systems, as well as friendly bacteria, usually keep *C. difficile* in check. At highest risk are elderly people and those who have chronic kidney disease or are taking antibiotics or medications that suppress the immune system. In such people, the bacterium produces a toxin

DIARRHEA RED FLAGS: WHEN TO SEEK IMMEDIATE TREATMENT

Diarrhea symptoms are nearly always unpleasant and uncomfortable, but it is important to know when you need to get urgent medical assistance. If you have any of the following symptoms, call your doctor right away:

- Severe abdominal pain
- Sudden onset of abdominal pain
- Sudden onset of sustained (more than several hours) nausea and vomiting
- New onset of having five to ten bowel movements a day

The following diarrhea symptoms are less urgent but also are red flags for medical attention soon:

- Blood in the stool
- Fever with diarrhea
- Loss of appetite with diarrhea
- Weight loss of more than five to ten pounds as the result of diarrhea
- Recurrent abdominal pain that lasts more than four to six hours
- Anemia

that severely damages the lining of the colon (large bowel, where stool is stored) so that it does not absorb fluid, causing cramping, diarrhea, and high fever. In weak or elderly people, the disease can be fatal. Among healthy adults not in the hospital, only 3 percent harbor the organism. (Please see the "Red Flags" sidebar for more about diarrhea symptoms that require immediate treatment.)

Chronic Conditions and Diseases

Several diseases and disorders can either cause diarrhea or make it worse.

Irritable Bowel Syndrome (IBS). This is not one condition, but rather a group of disorders affecting the large bowel (where stool is stored). Symptoms may include abdominal pain or discomfort, cramps, bloating, gas, diarrhea, or constipation. IBS is not a *structural* disease (meaning something is wrong with the bowel structure), but a *functional* disorder, meaning that the movement of food and fluids in the bowel is disrupted. Eighty percent of IBS patients are pre-menopausal women, and it is suspected that hormonal imbalances are at least in part responsible for disruptions in bowel functions in these women, either speeding up the movement of food and fluids, which causes diarrhea, or slowing them down, which causes con-

SYMPTOMS AND DIAGNOSIS OF IRRITABLE BOWEL SYNDROME

In the absence of "red flag" symptoms of diarrhea, the following symptoms—if they have persisted for three months, even "on and off"—are indications of IBS:

- Abdominal pain
- Stool changes in either consistency or frequency
- Absence of bowel movements during the evening
- Feeling of incomplete evacuation ("emptying") after a bowel movement
- Pain before a bowel movement and often relieved by it
- Increased mucus in stool

In order to diagnose IBS, your doctor will ask you to describe the timing, duration, and exact details of your symptoms, including type of pain, frequency, and type of bowel movements, as well as your medical history, to find out if your symptoms are consistent with those of the disorder. The Food and Symptom Log that you began in week one of this program will be a valuable resource for both you and your doctor as you demystify your diarrhea condition.

stipation. Both are symptoms of irritable bowel syndrome. (Please see the sidebar for diagnostic information about IBS.)

Crohn's Disease and Ulcerative Colitis. These are inflammatory bowel diseases that are far less common than IBS and are caused by a genetic predisposition, although the symptoms may resemble IBS. They are usually triggered by some event (such as a viral or bacterial enteritis, or a medication) that irritates the bowel, causing an inflammation. In people with these diseases, the response to the trigger is exaggerated: the inflammatory response is severe, causing pain and diarrhea; moreover, there is no "shutoff" switch, so the inflammation continues even after the trigger has been eliminated,

SYMPTOMS AND DIAGNOSIS OF CROHN'S AND ULCERATIVE COLITIS

Crohn's often "masquerades" as IBS, because it has similar symptoms. However, people with ulcerative colitis and Crohn's disease may experience more severe pain, as well as bleeding during bowel movements. While the symptoms of IBS and Crohn's are similar, certain tests may reveal abnormalities that are present in Crohn's disease but not in IBS. Your doctor will perform these tests if indicated. If Crohn's is suspected, for example, your doctor will likely do the following:

- Take a complete medical history, including all of your symptoms of cramps and diarrhea
- Perform a physical exam in order to detect whether you are having pain in your abdomen
- Order an endoscopy (in which a tube is inserted through the colon [large bowel] that allows the doctor to see inside the colon), and possibly x-rays, to detect abnormalities such as ulcers or inflammation inside the colon and small bowel
- Biopsy tissue from your intestines

resulting in continuing damage to the lining of the intestine and altering both the absorption and secretion of fluids by the intestine. Crohn's disease can involve both the small bowel and colon, whereas ulcerative colitis involves only the colon. Both can cause inflammation of the colon resulting in diarrhea. These disorders are often differentiated by medical tests. For this reason, Crohn's and ulcerative colitis are called *self-perpetuating disorders*, and they must be diagnosed by a thorough evaluation. Both of these conditions can masquerade as irritable bowel, so it is important to seek medical help and a proper diagnosis.

Celiac Sprue. This condition is due to a gluten intolerance that affects the lining of the small bowel and changes the way in which your body processes and absorbs food and fluids. (Gluten is found in wheat, rye, barley, and many other grains.) This disease is caused by a genetic predisposition and is common among people with Irish or European ancestry. For people with celiac sprue, gluten is not fully broken down during digestion, and the leftover "unbroken" parts of the grain stimulate the lining cells of the gut to overreact, causing inflammation and altered function. These changes in the lining of the gut mean that food nutrients don't get fully absorbed, possibly causing anemia (iron deficiency) and bone problems from decreased absorption of calcium. Please see Chapter 6 for details about diagnosing and managing gluten intolerance.

Diabetes. Diabetes can cause diarrhea in several ways:

■ Insulin is necessary to drive the glucose—sugar in food absorbed from the small intestine—to the blood and then into the cells of the body. Problems with insulin production, as occur in diabetes, lead to the incomplete usage of glucose in individual cells throughout the body. This causes the level of blood sugar to rise, which then brings on other problems, as itemized in the following entries. In addition, diabetes can impair the normal movement of food and fluid through the intestine, causing diarrhea. (Please see

Chapter 7 for more details about the digestive problems associated with this condition.)

■ Dietetic and so-called sugarless foods may contain large amounts of sorbitol and other sugar alcohols, which are potent laxatives.

■ About 5 percent of people with diabetes also develop celiac sprue (gluten intolerance).

■ People with diabetes often have problems with the pancreas, which lead to a decreased ability to properly digest food.

■ Diabetes may give rise to large numbers of bacteria in the small bowel, interfering with digestion and the absorption of food.

Overactive Thyroid. This condition can cause weight loss, increased nervousness, and intolerance to heat. When you are very hot, your pores open, you sweat more, and your body "speeds up" and metabolizes faster. It also speeds up the bowel, which causes diarrhea.

Diverticular Disease. This disease of the colon, which affects up to 20 percent of people over age fifty, may resemble irritable bowel. It is due to thickening of the muscles of the colon, which causes increased pressure. In turn, the thickening results in several diverticula that are little sacs in the wall of the colon. Diverticular disease causes symptoms that include intermittent episodes of diarrhea, straining before a bowel movement, pencil-thin stools, and pain that is relieved after a bowel movement.

Surgery

Abdominal surgery can transform the way your digestive system works. Diarrhea may result when segments of the small bowel are removed (for example, as a treatment for Crohn's disease or because of a blood clot). Surgical removal of the gallbladder may also result in diarrhea, since the bile that it normally stores, which helps you digest a meal, remains in the intestines for a longer period than normal, stimulating your large bowel to produce more fluids and causing diarrhea.

Antibiotics and Other Medications

Your bowel contains billions of bacteria, and when you eat, the "good" bacteria in your gut can help to break down the food so that its nutrients can be digested and absorbed. If you need to take antibiotics to battle an infection, the medicine may also knock out these helpful digestive bacteria. As a consequence, the sugars (from carbohydrates) and cellulose (from vegetables) in your food are not properly broken down during the digestive process. The by-products accumulate in your small and large bowel and stimulate the lining to put out more fluid, and this can result in diarrhea.

In addition to antibiotics, other medications, including antacids, diuretics, and antigout medications such as colchicine, can accelerate the speed at which food and fluid pass through your body, causing diarrhea. Be sure to ask your doctor about the side effects of medications that affect digestion or absorption of nutrients from food.

Eating Disorders

If you have an eating disorder, especially if it involves the overuse of laxatives (which are prescribed only to alleviate constipation) or diuretics (which make your body lose water), please discuss this fact with your doctor. Using laxatives or any medication when they are not prescribed can invite serious health problems.

▶Diarrhea Food and Drink Culprits

Some of the snacks you pop into your mouth without thinking may be a major source of your problem. If you consume large quantities of foods rich in sugars such as fructose and sorbitol, you may have *osmotic diarrhea*, which means that the sugars actually pull fluid

LAXATIVE FOOD AND DRINK ALERTS

No matter what is causing your diarrhea, certain foods and beverages will likely make it worse:

- Fruits—especially peaches, pears, cherries, apples, orange juice, and apple juice, which contain large amounts of fructose and sorbitol; unripe fruits can also be problematic
- Brassica vegetables—such as broccoli, asparagus, cauliflower, brussels sprouts, and cabbage
- Beans
- Coffee
- Any foods left unrefrigerated—especially egg salad, potato salad, and custards
- Milk products—among people who are lactose intolerant
- Sorbitol-rich foods—which include nearly all products that claim to be "sugar free," especially diabetic jams, ice creams, candies, and similar foods (Read labels carefully!)
- Colas—sixteen ounces of a cola beverage contains forty grams of fructose, and this sugar is not well absorbed in about 15 percent of healthy people and can contribute to diarrhea
- Candy bars—these and other sugar-rich foods in large quantities increase the sugar load in your intestines and can cause diarrhea

into the bowel. Watch out for those so-called sugarless mints and gums, since they are not actually free of sugar at all! Rather, they contain hard-to-digest sugars such as sorbitol—a type of sugar alcohol, which is a potent laxative. All "sugarless" gums contain one to two grams of sorbitol per piece, and as little as five grams of sorbitol can cause diarrhea. This and similar sugar alcohols are the main ingredients in many "sugarless" products.

I have had patients who tended to chew sugarless gum all day long or regularly snack on sugarless candies. When they stop, so does the diarrhea. Sorbitol also occurs naturally in many fruits, which is why it is wise to moderate your consumption of fruit while trying to control diarrhea.

Diarrhea can also result from food intolerances and sensitivities. If you have food intolerances, the partially digested sugars and cellulose fibers are not fully broken down by bacteria, and the remaining breakdown products can irritate the bowel lining, stimulating the production of fluid and causing cramps and loose stools. People who are lactose intolerant, for example, cannot fully digest the sugar (lactose) in milk and dairy products, causing diarrhea. (See Figure 2.2.) Vegetarians, if they eat a large amount of fiber, often have a similar inability to fully digest vegetables, beans, and other cellulose-rich foods. The "Laxative Food and Drink Alerts" sidebar itemizes specific foods that may be causing you problems.

Strategies to Slow the Flow

As you can see, many factors can change the way in which your digestive system functions. Whether your problem is diet or disease, the food and fluids you consume can have a major impact. Even if you have a medical disorder, prevention of diarrhea is largely a matter of common sense. If certain foods give your intestinal tract a hard time, *stay away from them*. Despite the long list of problem foods, there are plenty of other strategies you can use to defend your gut against diarrhea that is caused by bacteria:

- Check expiration dates.
- Wash all fruits and vegetables well.
- Rinse chicken before you cook it.
- Cook chicken and other meats fully, and serve all cooked food piping hot.
- Clean all food preparation areas such as countertops and cutting boards with soap and hot water.
- Wash your hands thoroughly before and after handling food.

Figure 2.2 **Normal Lactose Digestion Versus Lactose Intolerance**

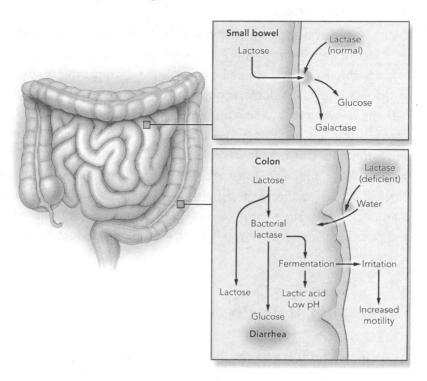

If you are lactose intolerant, you have trouble fully digesting the sugar (lactose) that is in milk and other dairy products, and this can cause diarrhea. The top diagram shows the lactose getting broken down normally in the small bowel. The bottom diagram shows what happens in people who are lactose intolerant: the incompletely digested lactose goes into the lower part of the large bowel, where it causes irritation and increased fluid release, and this can result in abdominal cramps, bloating, and diarrhea ("increased motility").

- Be careful about eating foods left outside for a long time at barbecues or picnics, and beware of street vendors, for the same reason. Bacteria can grow easily in the warm air. Don't take home leftovers from these sources.
- Even indoors, leftovers should be refrigerated quickly after the meal.
- Consult your log to narrow down which food may have given you a particular bout of diarrhea.

FECAL INCONTINENCE: A DIFFICULT BUT IMPORTANT TOPIC

I am amazed at how often physicians fail to ask their patients about fecal incontinence—losing stool in the underwear or before making it to the bathroom. This is a repellent and embarrassing topic for people to discuss with their doctors, but it must not be overlooked. Most patients are reluctant to say they are losing control of their stool. To finesse the plain truth, they will often say they are having diarrhea and hope their doctor will prescribe a medicine that will control the incontinence. Stool incontinence can be a warning sign for other maladies, including diabetes. It can also be corrected through methods that include retraining the floor muscles of the pelvis with exercises and possible surgery. So, if you have this problem, be sure to discuss it with your doctor.

Foods That Help Prevent Diarrhea

As you cut out problem foods and "diarrhea culprits," you can substitute the following foods to soothe your irritated bowel: white rice; white bread; bananas; potatoes; and well-cooked fish, chicken, broiled meats, and veal. These foods help because they do not contain a lot of fiber, which absorbs fluid like a sponge and holds it in the bowel, speeding up the digestion process. This regimen should be followed only on a temporary basis, until your digestion is stable. Your goal should be to have a balanced diet that includes fiber-rich foods such as vegetables, fruits, and whole grains, as well as healthy proteins.

Your Four-Week Plan for Diarrhea

Now that you have a frame of reference for the causes and symptoms of diarrhea, as well as when to seek immediate treatment, you can launch your Four-Week Plan for relief. As you begin the

) SUGAR-FREE, NOT TROUBLE-FREE

Mary L., a twenty-eight-year-old woman, had been experiencing chronic diarrhea for three months and had not been able to identify the source. She had undergone numerous tests and tried every medicine, but nothing relieved her symptoms. At our first appointment, I noticed that she was chewing gum and asked how much gum she chewed every day. "I chew about two packs of sugarless gum a day," she told me. "I work at a fast-food restaurant, and if I ate all the food that is freely available, I'd gain ten to fifteen pounds, so I use sugarless gum and mints to avoid eating."

Together, Mary and I examined the label and saw that each piece of gum contained about two grams of sorbitol. As you now know, sorbitol and other sugar alcohols that are in "sugarless" gum are forms of carbohydrates that are poorly absorbed in the body and can cause diarrhea.

I suggested that Mary read labels carefully and cut all sugar alcohols and sorbitol-containing products—including gum and mints—out of her diet. Two months later, Mary's diarrhea symptoms had disappeared! But she had gained ten pounds. We discussed counting calories, reducing portion size, and exercising with daily weights to gradually lose weight (one to two pounds per week).

program, I suggest talking to your doctor, because a complete medical and dietary history will be integral in diagnosing the causes of your diarrhea. You should be prepared to supply your doctor with the answers to the following questions. If you are not sure of an answer, wait until you have recorded the details in your Food and Symptom Log during week one, and then share the information with your doctor.

- How much coffee, tea, or other caffeine-containing beverages do you drink every day?
- How many cola-type beverages do you drink?

- How many sorbitol-containing foods do you eat, and how often? (Read labels carefully to be sure.)
- How many candy bars and other sugar-rich foods do you eat every day?
- What dairy foods—such as milk, cheese, butter, ice cream, custards, and cream sauces—do you eat, and how often? Do you notice that they lead to diarrhea as well as gas, bloating, and cramps?
- Do you have an eating disorder, such as bulimia, or do you use laxatives? (It is essential to share this kind of information with your doctor.)
- Where have you traveled recently—especially foreign travel?

Week One

Start your Food and Symptom Log, and begin your detective work. As I cautioned in Chapter 1, you shouldn't change your eating habits this week, but your log must be all-inclusive. Be especially aware of your intake of the foods listed in the "Laxative Food and Drink Alerts" sidebar. Make sure to record absolutely everything, particularly all those incidentals such as candy, gum, and mints. As Mary L.'s story shows, those simple treats could easily be the main culprits behind your symptoms.

If you suspect that you are sensitive to lactose (or if you have another food sensitivity), always record in detail your intake of dairy products (or whichever food seems to give you trouble). When dining in restaurants or at friends' homes, make sure to ask if your meal is cooked in butter, or if there is milk or cheese in a sauce. Don't be shy! Most people are more than happy to tell you how things are cooked, especially if you explain that you have a sensitivity. Also record any vitamins, supplements, and medicines you are taking—they may well be affecting your symptoms.

Don't forget to log your symptoms as well as your food intake. This is the best way to figure out which foods trigger your symptoms. For more details about what you should be doing during this first week, refer back to Chapter 1.

) RECOMMENDED READING

Many chewing gums and mints contain significant amounts of sorbitol and sugar alcohols that are not absorbed into your body but can cause diarrhea.

- For more of the skinny about sorbitol and other fruit alcohols, visit caloriecontrol.org/sorbitol.html.
- An article in the January 12, 2008, issue of the *British Medical Journal* observed the negative consequences of sugarless gum. The observation done by Dr. Herbert Lochs and Dr. Juergen Bauditz described two patients who experienced rapid weight loss due to excessive diarrhea caused by sugarless gum.

Week Two

Now it's time to analyze the way you eat. Continue your log, and see if you can detect a pattern developing. Don't change your diet yet, but do start thinking about which factors tie your food and symptoms together. Week two is all about changing your eating habits without altering your diet. This is particularly important if you suffer from chronic diarrhea, as your portion sizes and the speed at which you eat can certainly affect what happens on the other end. Refer back to Chapter 1 for information about how to change your eating habits. Think of this week as a deep breath and a chance to relax; enjoy your meals, rather than dreading that trip to the bathroom.

Week Three

It's time to take action! Review your log, and make a list of the foods, beverages, and supplements that appear to be linked to your symptoms. This week, you will eliminate or significantly decrease your intake of these foods. I repeat: *do not stop taking any prescription medication without talking to your doctor*. In particular, think about completely eliminating foods from the foregoing

"Laxative Food and Drink Alerts" list. Every time you want to pop a sorbitol-filled mint into your mouth, think about how wonderful you will feel when you are diarrhea free. It can be tricky to eliminate lactose if you are newly lactose intolerant, but view it as an opportunity to explore all the nondairy options available. A scoop of ice cream isn't worth being trapped in the bathroom for the greater part of your day. Refer back to Chapter 1 to learn about the "ABAB" system you should be using this week.

If you think that more than one food is causing your symptoms, test this hypothesis by eliminating foods one at a time and recording the results. In such situations, it is perfectly fine to extend this part of the plan beyond one week in order to complete a thorough analysis of your problem foods.

Week Four

This week, you will begin reintroducing the foods that you eliminated during week three. Again, if more than one food is involved, reintroduce them one at a time. Keep up your log, and dutifully document everything you are eating, as well as your symptoms. You will become aware of which foods seem to act as laxatives and aggravate your symptoms. It is all right if this process takes more than one week, especially if you are working with multiple foods. Give your body enough time to react to each reintroduced item. This is also a good time to discuss your progress with your doctor, nutritionist, or dietitian if you have questions about your new diet and new lifestyle.

Chapter 3

Constipation

I f you are suffering from constipation, you are not alone; it is one of the most common digestion problems, affecting 15 to 20 percent of the population throughout the world, and women more frequently than men. Constipation can take several forms: you may not be having enough bowel movements and you feel bloated and uncomfortable; you may be having dry and hard bowel movements that are difficult or even painful to pass; or you may be in the grips of both conditions.

Let us imagine for a moment that you are walking into my office seeking help for these problems. Constipation is disrupting your days and nights with abdominal pain, bloating, or discomfort. You may not have been able to pass a bowel movement in two or three days or even a week, and you are frustrated. You just want to get on with your life. If these symptoms have been going on for a month or more, you can assume you have chronic constipation. Competing advertisements are trying to sell you over-the-counter medications, all of which claim to hold the secret to a constipation-free life. You may have tried some of them, and perhaps they have worked temporarily, but so far you have not found lasting relief.

When you enter my office, what you know for sure is that you are uncomfortable and that you need some way to get things moving. You may not know whether you have chronic constipation, or even what that really means. Dietary changes alone can help about 30

percent of sufferers. For others, a diagnosis of chronic constipation means that some interventions might be necessary, including
the use of bulking agents. These treatments for chronic constipation are described later in the chapter. You also may not know that
there could be many causes behind your constipation, or how to
approach the problem. This chapter will help you understand the
causes of your constipation, give you some discussion points to use
with your doctor, and arm you with strategies to help gain relief.

▶What Is Constipation?

You probably know about many of the symptoms of constipation,
but you may not have a practical standpoint from which to analyze your condition. Typically, a healthy person will have a bowel
movement from one to three times a day, but at least once every
three days. Constipation is commonly defined as fewer than three
bowel movements per week, but this is not a complete descrip-
tion. Constipation can also cause changed consistency of stools
(for example, more than 25 percent of your stools are hard and
are difficult to pass) and difficulty passing bowel movements: you
may continue to have bowel movements every day, but they may be
painful, and you might experience a feeling of incomplete evacuation. You might also feel as though there is something blocking the
flow of stool, and you might sometimes have to resort to manual
maneuvers to help get things out. Any of these symptoms may indicate that you have chronic constipation.

While constipation caused by disease is beyond the scope of
this book, several conditions may either trigger constipation or
make it worse. In general, there are two types of constipation
that are not caused by a specific, underlying disease or condition:
slow-transit constipation and dyssynergic-response constipation.
While neither type is serious, both can be bothersome, and both
can be effectively treated and brought under control. Some people
actually have both kinds of constipation, and your doctor can use

certain tests to identify which kind you have and recommend corresponding treatments. I'll expand on these a little later in this chapter.

Slow-Transit Constipation

Also called *generalized colon inertia*, this is the most common type of constipation, affecting about 5 percent of the population. It occurs when the muscles throughout the colon—not just on the pelvic floor, as in dyssynergic response—have slowed, making it more difficult to move stool out of the colon. It can be present from adolescence onward and also be caused by aging, eating less, dietary changes (see "Constipation Food and Drink Culprits" later in this chapter), medication, pregnancy, childbirth, or hysterectomy. All of these factors can affect the muscle functioning of the entire colon.

Dyssynergic-Response Constipation

This disorder affects only the muscles of the pelvic floor—as opposed to the entire colon—and can be caused by childbirth or hysterectomy, as well as growing older. Dyssynergic-response constipation happens when your colon becomes a little "confused" and the pelvic floor muscles do not work in a coordinated fashion. Normally, when the brain gets a signal that the colon and rectum are full of stool, it responds by sending nerve signals to contract the pelvic muscles and relax the muscles of the anus. This correct sequence of events causes muscles to push the stool toward the rectum at just the right angle. At the same time, the lowermost rectal muscles relax, allowing the stool to pass out of the anus. Think of a tube of toothpaste: you remove the cap and squeeze the tube, and the toothpaste comes out easily.

With dyssynergic response, the signaling process goes awry: the upper muscles relax, while the muscles near the rectum contract. As you can imagine, this makes it difficult and often painful to move stool out of the colon. In our toothpaste analogy, think of the cap as still on the tube.

What Causes Constipation?

Looking beyond the two main types of constipation, individual and sometimes elusive factors may be behind your symptoms. Before getting to the foods that can aggravate or ameliorate your condition, let's investigate some of the other causes.

Not Enough Fluids

You may be hearing a lot these days about the importance of drinking water. When it comes to constipation, those eight to ten glasses of water or other fluids (a minimum of one and a half quarts) per day are crucial to maintaining a healthy digestive system and avoiding constipation. If you don't give your body enough fluid, things just won't flow. You don't have to restrict yourself to drinking only blah water, though: almost any beverage will help do the trick! Are you a big fan of coffee? Step right up. Caffeinated beverages such as coffee and tea do a good job of stimulating the bowel, which can ease some of the symptoms of constipation.

Underactive Thyroid

When the thyroid is healthy, it produces hormones that facilitate and accelerate in a normal fashion all of the processes within your body. These include your heart rate, blood flow, and contraction of the muscles in your small and large intestine. All of these processes slow down if your thyroid isn't functioning at the optimal level. This will make you feel sluggish and tired, both outside and in. As you might guess, a slowed digestive system can easily lead to constipation. Your doctor can test and prescribe treatment for underactive thyroid.

Diabetes

As I explained in the previous chapter, diabetes has many effects on digestion, one of which is slow stomach or gastric emptying (*gastroparesis*), meaning that the process of moving food and waste along the bowel is sluggish, causing constipation, as well as dyspepsia, nausea, vomiting, and bloating. If you have diabetes and are constipated, you should discuss remedies with your doctor, as well as following the dietary strategies in this book. (Please see Chapter 7 for details about digestion problems associated with this disease.)

Irritable Bowel Syndrome

Also as mentioned in Chapter 2, irritable bowel syndrome is a group of disorders affecting the large bowel, which is where stool is stored. IBS can cause both diarrhea and constipation and is especially prevalent in premenopausal women. In the case of constipation, it appears that hormonal imbalances can disrupt bowel function by slowing the movement of food and fluids. If you are concerned that your symptoms may be caused by IBS, please turn back to the "Symptoms and Diagnosis of Irritable Bowel Syndrome" sidebar in Chapter 2 for diagnostic information, and discuss the remedies with your doctor.

Medications

Many over-the-counter medications, such as those to treat allergies, can give you constipation by slowing down the colon. If you are taking any of the medications in the following list, ask your doctor if they could be a part of your problem. If so, you might be advised to take a stool softener while you are on these kinds of drugs. This is only a temporary treatment, however. Far more effective are wise food choices and drinking enough fluids. These medications include:

- Antihistamines
- Tricyclic antidepressants
- Calcium carbonate and other calcium products used to maintain bone health
- Calcium channel blockers (used to treat high blood pressure)
- All narcotics, especially derivatives of codeine such as Percocet, Vicodin, Oxycontin, and oxycodone
- Antidiarrheal drugs, such as Imodium and Lomotil—which can cause rebound constipation

Basically, anything that interferes with the way your body processes food and fluids can influence your digestive system. As you build your Four-Week Plan, remember to include all medications in your approach. Ask your doctor about their potential digestive side effects, and weigh the fact that these drugs may be causing some of your symptoms. Reiterating my earlier caveat: *make sure you consult with your doctor before stopping any prescription medications.*

Low Potassium and Magnesium

Having insufficient levels of potassium and magnesium in your bloodstream may interfere with the way muscles work in the small bowel and colon. The muscles that are supposed to contract in order to control the movement of stool may not be doing their jobs of propelling the contents of the bowel along the gastrointestinal tract. Low potassium and magnesium levels are usually *not* the result of your diet, unless you have a condition such as celiac sprue (gluten intolerance, which is the subject of Chapter 6). Usually, these deficiencies are caused by medications, such as diuretics or laxatives, especially if you are self-prescribing them without a doctor's supervision—something that I strongly discourage. Your doctor can test for these conditions and prescribe appropriate treatments.

While diet, as noted, is usually not at the root of the problem, you should be aware that bananas, oranges, cantaloupe, strawberries, and potatoes are potassium-rich foods, as is the herb turmeric. Magnesium-rich foods include black beans, whole-grain cereals, raw broccoli, halibut, and nuts.

Hysterectomy

Statistics show that about 5 percent of women who have had hysterectomies experience constipation that is difficult to manage. If you notice a new onset or a worsening of constipation symptoms after a hysterectomy, be sure to let your doctor know. The suggestions in this chapter should also yield some relief.

CONSTIPATION RED FLAGS: WHEN TO SEEK IMMEDIATE TREATMENT

Constipation is never easy, but there are times when it may be connected with something more serious. It's important to know when your symptoms could be dangerous and require urgent medical attention. If you have any of the following symptoms, call your doctor promptly. The term *new onset* refers to a variable time period ranging from one to four weeks.

- New onset of constipation after age forty-five; this may be a sign of colon cancer
- Constipation accompanied by sudden changes in bowel habits, especially sudden decreased frequency of bowel movements
- Passing pencil-thin stools
- Unintentional significant weight loss: more than ten pounds in one to two months
- Decreased appetite
- Red blood in the stool
- New development of anemia
- New difficulty passing a bowel movement, with persistent pain in the lower abdomen

Other Disease-Related Causes

Certain other conditions can lead to constipation or make it worse. If you have multiple sclerosis (MS) or Parkinson's disease, in particular, you may be at a higher risk for constipation symptoms. Some of the medications used for these conditions may have constipating side effects. In addition, lack of physical exercise may make constipation worse in individuals with MS or Parkinson's. Physical exercise is a good idea for everyone and benefits digestion, and the sedentary lifestyles that often accompany these diseases, along with effects on the nervous system, increase the risk of constipation.

▶ Constipation Food and Drink Culprits

As you begin to work on your Four-Week Plan, remember that our diets consist of a balance of "laxative" foods, those that tend to facilitate bowel movements, and "constipating" foods, those that slow the bowels. You are what you eat, and your bowel movements reflect your diet, absent any of the underlying conditions discussed earlier. If your diet contains an excessive amount of the following foods without a balance, it can tend to bind you up:

- Rice, especially white rice
- White bread
- Potatoes
- Fish
- Chicken
- Turkey
- Beef

Limiting the intake of fruits, grains, and vegetables and drinking less than one quart of total fluid per day can contribute to constipation. Always record any consumption of these foods in your Food and Symptom Log, and specify how much of them you eat. These foods, while excellent in the prevention of diarrhea, can significantly affect your constipation symptoms. Work on deleting these foods one at a time so that you can gauge the effect each one has on your digestive system, and/or add "laxative-type foods."

Remember that your symptoms are easily aggravated when you don't drink enough fluids. As you work on your log, see whether you are faithfully drinking eight to ten glasses of water or other beverages every day. That morning cup of coffee may actually relieve some of your discomfort! Does this seem like too much to drink? Try taking a water bottle or a thermos to work, and just keep refilling it throughout the day. You'll be surprised at how thirsty your body really is. Make coffee or tea dates with your friends—it's a made-in-the-shade way to get some bowel-easing fluid into your body while socializing!

Constipation Cures

Foods that may be terrible for people with one gastrointestinal condition can be extremely beneficial for other digestive problems. Many of the foods on the "culprit" list in the diarrhea chapter can alleviate some of your constipation symptoms. These laxative foods can help get your bowels moving in the right direction. As you examine your diet, check whether you are getting enough (or any!) of the following foods:

- Fruits—especially peaches, pears, cherries, apples, orange juice, and apple juice
- Brassica vegetables—such as broccoli, asparagus, cauliflower, brussels sprouts, and cabbage
- Beans
- Whole-grain breads
- Coffee
- Tea
- High-fiber foods—such as celery and salads

Of course, you don't want to overdo it with these foods; that can take you from one extreme to the other. Notwithstanding, these natural laxatives may help you on your path to a healthier digestive system. Think about creating a balance, rather than just overloading on natural laxatives.

Take the Natural Route

Chronic constipation is uncomfortable and disruptive to your everyday life. It may therefore be tempting to raid the shelves of your local pharmacy for every laxative you can grab. What you may not know is that these over-the-counter products can actually get in the way of your efforts to get your colon working.

Laxative medications can irritate your bowel and colon in order to stimulate their function. This is not how your body is supposed to work, and enough laxative use will actually change the way your colon and bowel respond to signals. They will become less likely to respond to normal, healthy stimuli, creating a dependence on laxative medications. As you continue to use these treatments, they will become less and less effective, as your digestive system will require higher and higher levels of irritation in order to function. Talk to your doctor before using laxatives, and try out some of the "natural laxatives" just listed before turning to over-the-counter medications.

If you don't move your bowels for three or more days and are still uncomfortable even after drinking a minimum of one and a half to two quarts of fluid a day and changing your diet, you can try the *occasional* stool softener, as well as laxatives such as Miralax or milk of magnesia or bulking agents such as Metamucil, always in consultation with your doctor. These medications ordinarily should not become a long-term treatment for chronic constipation.

▶The Four-Week Plan: Putting Your Knowledge to Work

Now it's time to design and implement your individualized Four-Week Plan. Look back at Chapter 1 for some ideas about how to get started. The Four-Week Plan will allow you to answer them and to find some digestive relief.

Don't forget that you should not change your diet at all during the first week; just keep track of everything that goes into your mouth, and make sure to note your symptoms as well. Don't be afraid to ask questions about your meal if someone else prepared it; think of it as part of your detective work!

As you begin to change your eating habits and diet, use the list of constipation culprits to get some ideas about which foods may be hindering you on your journey to digestive health. If you have questions, or if you aren't sure about the linkage between a certain food and your symptoms, don't hesitate to ask your doctor for help. The constipation Four-Week Plan is targeted to creating a balance between laxative foods and nonlaxative foods; you may end up doing more *adding* than *eliminating* as you gain control of your condition. Your log may show you that you just need to add a few more glasses of water and an extra salad or two to your diet!

Four Weeks Later and No Relief in Sight?

While a diet transformation may relieve your symptoms to some degree, there are times when that just isn't enough. Since constipation can be traced to more than one contributor, there are situations in which additional treatment may be necessary. If your symptoms haven't improved after you've worked on your diet, talk to your doctor. Your doctor will want to know whether you have one of the underlying conditions discussed earlier, as well as whether you have slow-transit or dyssynergic-response constipation. As you are now fully aware, medications, underactive thyroid, diabetes, hysterectomy, multiple sclerosis, and Parkinson's, as well as eating less than normal (decreased dietary intake), can all make constipation symptoms worse. When you do meet with your doctor, here is a list of the kind of information you should be ready to provide:

What to Tell Your Doctor—Discussion Points
- How frequently do you move your bowels? Do you feel pain, bloating, or other symptoms? Does the menstrual cycle affect your bowel movements? In this regard menses frequently leads to increased stool frequency in women.
- How is constipation affecting your life?
- Where are you having the most discomfort? You are probably having stomach pain, but where is it located: below or above your belly button? Below is usually a problem with the colon, whereas pain above the belly button is less likely to be

related to constipation, signifying a problem with the small bowel, stomach, pancreas, or gallbladder. Constipation usually causes abdominal discomfort lower down. Be sure to explain the location and duration of pain to your doctor, what brings it on, what relieves it, and what other symptoms you experience, such as bloating or distension.

- What foods do you eat a lot of? In particular, does your diet contain adequate amounts of fruit, vegetables, and whole-grain foods?
- How much water and other beverages do you drink? In particular, are you drinking at least a quart of fluid a day?
- Are you on any medications, such as antihistamines, pain medications, or high blood pressure medicine?
- Are you having unusual weight gain or loss?
- How does your menstrual cycle affect bowel movements?
- Have you had a recent hysterectomy? (This procedure causes difficult-to-manage constipation in 5 percent of women.)

Cures for Chronic Constipation

If you have any of the conditions set forth in this chapter, your doctor can propose various treatments. For example, there is a simple way to test for slow-transit constipation, which can often be treated easily as well. I have my patients swallow "sitz markers," which are basically small, radiopaque (meaning they show up on x-rays) disks, right after they have had a bowel movement. I then perform an x-ray five days later to see where the sitz markers have gone. In a person with a normally functioning digestive system, the markers will no longer be in the body. By contrast, if most of the markers remain scattered throughout the colon, it means that the patient has slow-transit constipation. (See Figure 3.1.) The bottom diagram shows dyssynergic-type constipation where the pellets are concentrated in the lower most parts of the colon.

Once slow-transit constipation has been identified, I normally prescribe a bulking agent such as Metamucil. Bulking agents act

Figure 3.1 **Diagnosing Constipation with Sitz Markers**

Generalized Colonic Slowing

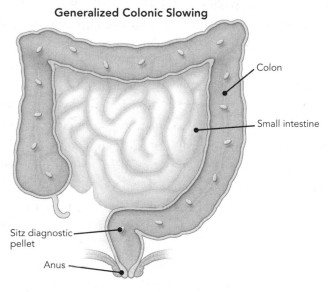

Colon

Small intestine

Sitz diagnostic pellet

Anus

Pelvic Floor Muscle Dysfunction

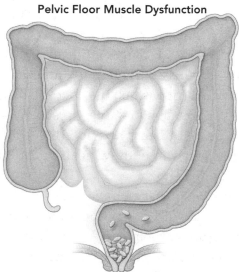

As part of the diagnostic evaluation for constipation, your doctor may prescribe a sitz marker study, in which you swallow tiny pellets that can be seen clearly on an x-ray. Five to seven days later, the x-ray will show how far they have progressed. (Normally, they should all have been eliminated by this time.) In the top diagram, they are scattered throughout the large bowel, indicating a generalized slowing of the colon. In the bottom diagram, they are concentrated in the lowermost part of the colon, indicating dyssynergic-response constipation: the pelvic floor muscles are not working in a coordinated fashion.

like little sponges, drawing fluid into the bowel and allowing the body to produce more frequent, bulkier stools. Why do you want a bulkier stool? Believe it or not, small stools are far more difficult to push out, as they do not stretch the walls of the rectum enough to facilitate passage. The spongelike function of bulking agents makes it much easier for the digestive muscles to do their jobs.

Testing for the other type of constipation, dyssynergic response, often requires special studies of how the muscles work—called anal/rectal motility. One example is defecography, in which barium is inserted into the rectum to see how well it empties. Anal/rectal motility studies may also involve putting a probe into the rectum to determine whether the muscles of the upper rectum that control defecation are acting in concert with the muscles of the lower rectum.

If you have dyssynergic-response constipation, you will usually be advised to undertake exercises that retrain your pelvic floor muscles to contract and release in the proper order. This is usually done using *biofeedback*, which gives you an awareness of bodily functions that usually occur automatically, such as heart rate and muscle contractions. This training is a painless—and often enlightening—experience during which the doctor will attach sensors to your skin and use a computer screen to show you changes in your muscle, brain wave, or heart activity. Biofeedback is one way to use your mind to help your body, which, come to think of it, is also the philosophy of this book!

A simple rule of digestion is that what goes in must come out—at least some of it. When the digestion process has extracted the proteins, vitamins, minerals, carbohydrates, fats, and other useful substances that serve as your body's fuel, the leftover waste products need to be eliminated, passing through your small and large intestines and, eventually, out through your colon and anus as a bowel movement. This chapter has shown how constipation interrupts this digestion process. While there are causes of constipation that may be beyond your control, you certainly have the power to improve your condition by changing what you eat and what—and how much—you drink.

KEEPING THINGS MOVING

Ellen G., thirty-eight, thought she was doing everything possible for good health. She had recently embarked on an intense exercise program, going to the gym five times a week for a vigorous, hour-long aerobic and weight-training workout. She was building muscles and stamina and losing weight. "I feel terrific after each workout," she told me. "Even though I am drenched in sweat, it feels good for my body."

Good, except for one problem: her lifelong pattern of infrequent bowel movements was getting worse. By the time she appeared in my office, she had been having only one bowel movement per week for the previous six months. When I questioned her about her digestive history, she told me that her usual pattern had been about three bowel movements per week, which were often hard and difficult to pass. "It was not good," she admitted, "but I had become used to it. But now, going only once a week is making me feel uncomfortable, heavy, and bloated."

Constipation can be defined as infrequent stools—two or fewer movements per week—or as stools that are consistently dry, hard, and difficult to pass. Ellen had both problems, and they were getting worse. My job was to work with her to figure out why and then advise her what to do about it.

While constipation can have numerous causes, each person typically has just a few main causes that interact. If we can identify them, the solution becomes fairly obvious. In Ellen's case, the first clue was the sweating. Constipation is a problem of too little fluid. (By contrast, diarrhea is a problem of too *much* fluid.) With the amount of fluid that Ellen was sweating out of her body almost every day, I wondered if she was replacing it by drinking enough water. Normally, I advise people to drink at least eight glasses of water a day. Other beverages, such as coffee, tea, or juices, will also help, but water is the most important.

Ellen, however, was simply not drinking enough to compensate for the amount of water she was losing through her copious sweating at the gym. "I just don't think of it," she explained. "I do stop at the water fountain at the gym periodically, but when I'm at work, I hardly h[...] time to drink!" To solve this problem, Ellen agreed to buy a t[...] ounce plastic water bottle (making sure it was made of saf[...]

material) and keep it with her, sipping regularly and refilling it four or five times a day. She takes it with her to the gym, and it has become a fixture on her desk at work.

There was more to Ellen's constipation problem than insufficient water, however. I also asked her to tell me what medications she was taking, and we discussed her dietary habits to boot. First, the medication: during the past six months, her doctor had started her on two new medications, a tricyclic antidepressant and an antihistamine for recurrent allergies. Both of these medications are known to slow down the bowel.

Then we turned to diet. Ellen had been keeping a Food and Symptom Log as part of her Four-Week Plan, so we reviewed it together. "I'm not seeing a lot of fruits and vegetables," I commented. "You are right," she conceded. "My habit is to eat more protein, because that is what I feel hungry for after a workout. I eat two protein bars a day and neglect fruits and vegetables!"

Remember that fiber-containing foods are critical to bowel health, and they can make an appreciable difference in constipation. Ellen and I came up with a new food plan for her. It featured whole-grain cereals or toast, along with at least one serving of fruit, for breakfast; a salad along with her protein for lunch; and at least one vegetable and a salad with her meat or fish for dinner. She was also going to include at least one serving of beans a day, in the form of a bean salad or Mexican refried beans, both of which are rich in fiber. During the day, instead of protein bars, she was to snack on apples, which are an excellent source of fiber as well as other nutrients. Throughout the day, she was also to make sure to drink at least two, and preferably three, quarts of fluid, especially during and after her workouts.

After just a few weeks, Ellen appeared in my office beaming. "I'm ... vel movement almost every day," she reported. "I ... re energetic, and I have even better workouts. The ... thought my depression was causing my constipa- ... en, in fact, it was the other way around. I'm feeling ... now that I told my doctor to wean me off of the

Chapter 4

Heartburn and Gastroesophageal Reflux Disease

You feel as if your chest is on fire. Antacids provide only a small amount of short-term relief before the pain returns with renewed ferocity. You can barely eat; you have trouble concentrating, meeting your daily responsibilities, and sleeping. *Heartburn* seems too mild a word to describe your suffering, and, in fact, it is. You may have gastroesophageal reflux disease, better known as GERD, and heartburn is one of the major symptoms.

GERD occurs when the food you eat, which is often mixed with digestive juices in the stomach, reverses direction, going "north" instead of "south" and passing back up into the esophagus, the tube that connects your mouth with your stomach, instead of continuing its downward journey into the small intestine. This happens when the muscles controlling the opening between the esophagus and the stomach do not work correctly. Called the esophageal sphincter, this circular band of tissue is at the base of the esophagus.

Normally, a certain amount of pressure holds the esophageal sphincter closed after food passes through it. If the sphincter relaxes at the wrong time, opening inappropriately after a meal, partially digested food may move back up into the esophagus.

The partially digested food that comes back up into the esophagus is called *refluxate*. Sometimes, this food can be acidic and cause a burning sensation, which is where the term *heartburn* comes from, even though it is not your heart that is "burning." The sensation usually begins as a burning feeling in the stomach that spreads up under the breastbone to the mid and upper chest. The pain may be triggered or made worse by bending over.

Some degree of reflux occurs in 95 percent of people after meals but is usually not associated with symptoms. About sixty million Americans, however, do have the bothersome or painful GERD symptoms just described. Of these, between 6 and 10 percent have some kind of symptom every day. So, there is a valid reason there are so many heartburn remedies advertised on television!

Our approach here will be different, however. We will use what I call "free therapy." These are dietary and behavioral practices that you can adopt without having to buy anything. In the event that these do not work, we will give other treatments their due later on in this chapter. First, let's take a closer look at GERD.

Symptoms of GERD and Heartburn

There is more to GERD than that familiar burning sensation. Here are some of the subtler symptoms:

- Frequent clearing of the throat
- Frequent coughing, including at night when you are lying down
- Hoarseness
- Feeling that something is sticking in your upper chest or throat as you are trying to swallow
- Chest pain that is not related to heart disease
- Asthma, bronchitis, or recurrent pneumonia
- Staining of your teeth or bad breath

Causes of GERD and Heartburn

Two factors contribute to GERD: the "doorway" between the stomach and the esophagus (esophageal sphincter) does not stay closed when it should; and the contents of the stomach (refluxate) are acidic. (See Figure 4.1.) If you feel this is happening to you, the sensible course is to discuss some of the possible causes, as listed in this section, with your doctor. In addition to these usual suspects, bending over or lifting heavy objects may make GERD sensations worse. Also, smoking can increase stomach acid as well as cause the esophageal sphincter to relax inappropriately, making the habit a GERD culprit on both counts. Yet another reason to quit!

Figure 4.1 **How GERD Causes "Burning"**

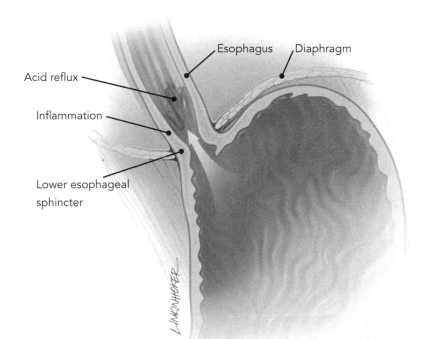

When the lower esophageal sphincter, the "doorway" between the stomach and the esophagus, relaxes and opens inappropriately, reflux can occur.

The Esophageal Sphincter Opens Inappropriately

There are several reasons why the "doorway" between the esophagus and the stomach may open at the wrong time. These include the following:

■ **Obesity.** Being overweight is a major risk factor for GERD, especially if your body mass index (BMI) is greater than 30. The BMI is calculated by determining weight in kilograms divided by height in meters squared. A normal BMI is less than 27. Stage 1 obesity is a BMI 30 to 35. Stage 2 is a BMI 36 to 40. Stage 3 or marked obesity is a BMI greater than 40. Being overweight is also defined if your waist measures more than forty inches if you're a male or more than thirty-five inches if you're a female. This puts added pressure on the sphincter muscles, making it more difficult for them to keep the "doorway" closed after you swallow food.

■ **Slow digestion.** Ideally, your stomach empties partially digested food as it is eaten, sending it down into the small bowel for further processing. If stomach emptying slows—also called delayed gastric emptying—either because of the high fat content of the food or as a result of conditions such as diabetes or certain drugs (see the following item), foods and liquids may remain in the stomach and then travel upward into the esophagus.

■ **Prescription and over-the-counter medicines.** Several drugs impede the action of the stomach and can cause delayed gastric emptying. These include antihistamines, calcium channel blockers and other blood pressure medications, tricyclic antidepressants, and antidiarrhea drugs.

■ **Pregnancy.** About 40 percent of women report reflux during all trimesters. The two principal reasons are that pregnancy puts greater pressure on the stomach, and the increased production of the hormone progesterone during pregnancy causes the esophageal sphincter muscle to relax.

Figure 4.2 **Hiatal Hernia**

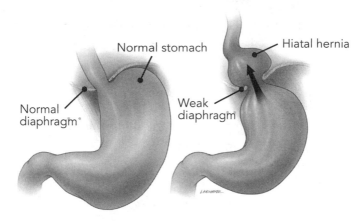

Hernias, such as this hiatal hernia at right, increase your risk of having GERD symptoms. In this image, protruding stomach tissue pushes against the esophageal sphincter, which causes acidic fluids from the stomach to remain in the esophagus for a longer period than normal. This can make GERD symptoms worse.

■ **Hiatal hernia.** A hernia is a condition in which one part of your body is protruding into another part where it does not belong, usually because of weakened tissues or too much pressure caused by exertion. With a hiatal hernia, part of the stomach has pushed through the diaphragm (a muscle that separates your chest cavity from your abdomen) at the opening where your esophagus joins your stomach. (Refer to Figure 4.2.) This protruding stomach tissue pushes against the esophageal sphincter, displacing it, and can either cause GERD or make it worse.

Acidic Stomach Contents

The burning sensation experienced during GERD derives from acidic stomach content, or refluxate. Consider these possible sources of that acidity:

■ **Not enough saliva.** You should be producing about a quart of saliva a day, one of the functions of which is to neutralize the

FOODS AND BEVERAGES THAT CAN CAUSE GERD SYMPTOMS

The following foods and beverages may cause or contribute to GERD. Consider eliminating them during week three to evaluate their effect on your symptoms.

Weakly Acidic Liquids
- Salad dressings or marinades containing vinegar
- Regular sugar-containing colas
- Orange and other citrus juices
- Tomato juice

Acidic Foods
- Citrus fruits
- Tomato-based foods such as spaghetti sauce and pizza
- Fatty foods
- Fried foods
- Garlic
- Onion

Foods and Liquids That Cause the Lower Esophageal Sphincter to Relax
- Chocolate
- Peppermint
- Caffeine

Other Causes
- Smoking

acid in your stomach. If you are not producing enough saliva, you might have a disorder of the salivary gland, or you might be taking medication that interferes with saliva production as one of its side effects. These medications include antihistamines, antidiarrheal drugs, and tricyclic antidepressants, to name a few.

■ **GERD culprits.** Regular cola beverages, orange juice, tomato juice, and salad dressings with vinegar are essentially weak acids and can cause GERD symptoms. Other acidic foods, especially citrus fruits, tomato-based foods such as spaghetti sauce and pizza, fried or fatty foods, and spicy foods, including garlic and onions, can also cause or contribute to GERD. Likewise, chocolate, beverages in addition to colas that contain caffeine or alcohol, and mint-flavored foods can all affect the nerves of the esophageal sphincter muscle, causing it to relax and allowing food to back up into the esophagus. The accompanying sidebar summarizes this "watch list."

Your Four-Week Plan for GERD and Heartburn

If you suspect that you have GERD, the first thing to do during week one is keep close track in your Food and Symptom Log of when you feel the related symptoms: After a meal? How long after? Related to any particular foods or beverages? Related to behaviors such as heavy lifting or bending over? This information will be useful when you meet with your doctor.

During week two, as you begin to modify your eating habits, pay particular attention to the following behaviors, which are related to GERD, and try to make the corresponding "free therapy" lifestyle changes:

■ If you have recently gained weight, even as little as ten pounds, take steps to lose it. Carrying those extra pounds can cause or contribute to GERD by increasing pressure on the stomach and increasing the likelihood of reflux. Weight loss often makes a significant difference in GERD symptoms because it reduces the pressure on the stomach.

■ Review with your doctor all of the medications you are taking, both over-the-counter and prescription. As previously noted, several common medications can cause or worsen GERD symptoms. *Do not stop taking any medications without consulting with your doctor!* You might want to ask about alternatives, however.

■ Avoid eating or drinking for three to four hours before you go to bed. Lying down before your stomach has emptied may cause reflux, because your stomach may still contain partially digested food and stomach acids, and by being in a horizontal position, you prevent gravity from doing its job of moving the food downward, where it belongs.

■ Do not smoke, but if you have not yet quit, definitely do not smoke after you eat. Obviously, this is easier to say than to do, but there are many excellent smoking-cessation programs, and I recommend asking your health-care provider for a referral.

■ Avoid wearing tight clothing that puts pressure on your stomach. This constriction may have the same effect as bending over and heavy lifting, putting pressure on the esophageal sphincter and causing stomach contents to back up into the esophagus.

■ During the night, it helps if your head, chest, and stomach are elevated, using the force of gravity to keep the stomach contents from moving upward. Raise the head of your bed by six to ten inches, using blocks. Do not merely increase the number of pillows, which will not work, because you are raising only your head, and you need to elevate your chest and stomach as well.

■ The position in which you sleep can also make a difference. Lying on your left side keeps your stomach in a dependent (lower) position, which decreases the likelihood of reflux.

During week three, the "food elimination" period, focus on the roster of GERD culprits previously cited. You can try cutting them out either one at a time or all at once, recording what happens. Whichever method you choose, reintroduce them one at a time dur-

RED FLAGS FOR GERD AND HEARTBURN

If your GERD symptoms are accompanied or characterized by any of the following, you should seek medical attention:

- Nausea and vomiting
- Difficulty or pain with swallowing
- Losing more than eight to ten pounds within three months
- Vomiting blood
- Duration of symptoms for more than ten years
- Symptoms that last longer than a few months and do not respond to dietary change or over-the-counter medicines such as Prilosec, Zantac, or Pepcid
- You are a Caucasian male over forty-five with GERD symptoms for ten years or longer—because of the risk for Barrett's esophagus, which is a precancerous condition
- Family history of either esophageal or stomach cancer

ing week four, and observe and record the results with precision. While you are doing this and avoiding acidic foods, you might want to increase your consumption of foods and beverages that soothe GERD and heartburn. These include yogurt, milk, ice cream, and smoothies. You might also try mashed potatoes, custards, and gelatin desserts, which are examples of foods that may be better tolerated. At this point, any nonirritating foods and foods that are not highly seasoned are safe to try. Avoid highly seasoned or spicy dishes.

Still Having Symptoms? Time for a Doctor Visit

If you have followed all of the dietary and behavioral changes—including losing weight and quitting smoking—and are still having symptoms, it is time to take yourself and your log to your doctor and ask for more help. This will, of course, lengthen your Four-Week Plan, but at least you will have determined that dietary and behavioral remedies are not helping you, and this information is useful for your doctor to have.

First, your doctor may wish to do some diagnostic testing. There are four tests that are generally used for GERD:

■ **Proton pump inhibitor.** A proton pump inhibitor is a type of drug that intercepts the final step in acid production by the stomach by blocking the pathway through which special cells in the stomach (parietal cells) produce acid. In the absence of red flags and under the supervision of a physician, this procedure involves two to four weeks of the administration of a medication such as Prilosec (omeprazole). If it leads to clear improvement, it serves as both a diagnostic test and appropriate treatment.

■ **Endoscopy and biopsy of the esophagus.** This procedure is recommended by a physician if red flags are present and/or symptoms persist despite treatment. It involves insertion of a tube that passes through the mouth to examine the esophagus, stomach, and upper small bowel, providing a direct look.

■ **Upper-gastrointestinal x-rays.** These diagnostic tools have been largely replaced by endoscopy when it is available. In certain circumstances, however, x-rays can provide additional useful information to your doctor.

■ **Twenty-four-hour esophageal pH study.** If GERD symptoms persist despite treatment, this procedure can determine whether you are experiencing acid reflux or nonacid reflux. Patients can have typical reflux symptoms even though acid production by the stomach is controlled, because of the reflux of nonacidic contents into the esophagus. This test tells the doctor whether the acid-suppressing medicines are working. You may still have nonacidic reflux, and you should make sure that you are adhering to the suggested lifestyle modifications. Even then, you may still have symptoms, and if so, you should discuss them with your doctor.

Depending on what these tests reveal, your doctor may recommend treatment. Possibilities include both medication and, in extreme cases, surgery.

Medical Treatments

Over-the-counter medicines, such as Tums and Maalox, as well as histamine H2 blockers (e.g., Zantac, Pepcid, Tagamet) and proton pump inhibitors (Prilosec) can be used on an as-needed basis to buffer the acid in your stomach. These drugs are most effective for mild symptoms. For more severe symptoms, your doctor may prescribe additional medication.

Proton pump inhibitors are a mainstay of long-term therapy. They are indicated in patients in whom an upper-gastrointestinal endoscopy has revealed evidence of inflammation in the lower esophagus, or to control persistent symptoms.

When All Else Fails: Surgery

Special types of surgery may be considered in selected patients for whom medical treatments have failed. The term *fundoplication* refers to surgery where the opening of the esophagus into the stomach is narrowed to bring about better control of reflux of stomach contents into the esophagus.

Summing Up

For most people, GERD and its accompanying symptoms, such as heartburn, are uncomfortable and bothersome but not life threatening. By following the four-week dietary and lifestyle plan in this chapter, many sufferers will find some relief. For those who do not, the medical and surgical therapies described have been found to be effective.

However, be aware that GERD symptoms can also be warning signs for more serious conditions that may lead to esophageal or stomach cancer. So, the main lesson of this chapter is that you must not ignore your symptoms. Try the Four-Week Plan, but if that does not work, or if you have any of the "red flag" warning symptoms, do not hesitate to contact your doctor for more detailed diagnosis and treatment.

SOOTHING THE BURN

For Andrea W., forty-four, over-the-counter liquid antacids had become her constant companion during the last several months. She sat in my office one late December, clearly uncomfortable, and described the burning sensation in the pit of her stomach that traveled under her breastbone. "I have pain most frequently after meals," she told me. "I can't concentrate on work or enjoy life anymore." The over-the-counter remedies provided only short-term relief before the pain returned. "At times, I feel as if the pit of my stomach and my chest are on fire," she said.

Andrea had a classic case of gastroesophageal reflux disease, the most common symptom of which is heartburn. Although she really did feel as if her heart was "burning," that is not what was going on. In actuality, the muscles controlling the opening between her stomach and her esophagus (the tubelike structure connecting the stomach with the mouth) were not working properly, and the opening to the stomach (called the esophageal sphincter) was not staying closed when it should, in order to keep the food in the stomach after it was swallowed. Instead, the sphincter was opening before the stomach had emptied, and the partially digested food, along with the digestive stomach acids, was backing up into the esophagus, traveling "north" toward the mouth instead of "south" toward the bowel.

As we talked, Andrea said she was well aware that certain foods and drinks aggravated the reflux. "Whenever I drink red wine, orange juice, or tomato juice, the symptoms get worse," she stated. "I also notice that even a simple salad causes heartburn if the dressing is very vinegary. Chocolate and peppermint also give me heartburn, and I've been trying to avoid all these things, as well as spicy foods, but there is only modest improvement."

With the persistence of her GERD symptoms, it was time for a detailed medical and dietary history. It turned out that over the past six months, Andrea had gained about fifteen pounds. "I got so busy at work that I wasn't eating very healthy food, and my exercise program slipped a bit," she said ruefully. "Also, this being the holiday season, it sure is easy to pack on the pounds at these parties!" Unknown to Andrea (and many other people!), gaining as little as ten pounds can put enough abdominal pressure on the stomach to cause the esophageal sphincter to open inappropriately. The flip side is that *losing* as little as ten pounds can notably improve GERD symptoms.

When I asked Andrea about any medications she was taking, she told me that her doctor had recently prescribed amitriptyline, a tricyclic antidepressant, which has several potential GERD-aggravating side effects. It tends to retard stomach emptying, causing the contents and acids to remain in the stomach longer than they should. It also cuts down on the production of saliva, which serves to neutralize stomach acids.

Now we had a plan of action: Andrea needed to lose fifteen pounds and talk to her doctor about changing to a different antidepressant with fewer gastrointestinal side effects. Hard as it was to lose the weight, Andrea was well motivated. "I was just tired of being in pain!" she told me. She lost the weight, changed her medication, and continued to watch for foods that stimulate GERD or make it worse. Within a few months, her symptoms had improved markedly, and she uses the over-the-counter antacids only sporadically, when she slips up on her diet.

Chapter 5

Dyspepsia

D octors use the word *dyspepsia* as a label for recurrent upper-abdominal discomfort that includes refluxlike symptoms, ulcerlike symptoms, and slow-stomach symptoms, all of which are described in this chapter. To lay the groundwork, let's first take a glance at a *non*medical definition of the word *dyspeptic*: "gloomy, pessimistic, and irritable," which might be a fitting way to describe your mood if you suffer regularly from heartburn, nausea, bloating, gas, and abdominal pain. It's a trial to remain upbeat when digestive discomfort is part of your daily routine, and dyspepsia is one of the most common digestive ailments. In fact, the term is used in reference to most gastrointestinal problems that occur as a result of food consumption, along with either structural or nonstructural problems of the digestive system.

Dyspepsia is actually a Greek word meaning "indigestion," encompassing the symptoms just cited as well as upper-abdominal discomfort. This discomfort is certainly reflected in the name of the ailment. Did you ever notice how many words describing problems start with the prefix *dys-*? This prefix indicates that whatever follows is not functioning properly. So, a diagnosis of dyspepsia means that your digestive system is somewhat—to use another *dys-* word—*dysfunctional*. This chapter addresses the wide variety of symptoms that get in the way of proper digestive function and cause dyspepsia.

▶Digestion by the Book

If you've been laid low by dyspepsia for a long time, it's probably hard to believe that it is even possible for a digestive system to function properly. Nevertheless, when dyspepsia is not getting in the way, your digestive system has the ability to operate like clockwork. The goal of this chapter (and of this book!) is to help you get your body back on track and remove the roadblocks to the proper flow of internal processes.

I described the gastrointestinal system in detail in the Introduction, so here is a "refresher course" that summarizes the main digestive functions: A healthy digestive system works through numerous steps to move food rapidly from your lips to your stomach and bowels. The first stage occurs in your mouth, where your teeth and saliva start breaking down the food. Next, it's off to the esophagus, which uses *peristalsis* to push the food down into the stomach. That is, the muscles of the esophagus contract and release to get the food moving through your body. Once the food makes it down to your stomach, it's time to mix it up. Digestive chemicals and stomach acids churn and mix with the partially digested food, breaking it down into much smaller pieces. This process, which takes a few hours, allows the digested food (now broken into much more manageable sizes) to move safely through the small and large intestines.

In the small intestine, tiny, hairlike projections called *villi* pull the nutrients out of the small particles of digested food and deliver those vital components to the bloodstream. This is a crucial aspect of digestion, as an unhealthy or malfunctioning small intestine can lead to severe malnourishment. (I'll talk more about this in the following chapter, in the context of how this digestive process is disrupted by celiac sprue.)

The food components that are not useful to your body keep traveling and move through the large intestine. Eventually, these waste products are pushed out of the body through the colon, leaving behind a healthy digestive system that is ready to absorb more nutrients. (For more about the colon, please see Chapter 3.)

▶Problems with Digestion

Now that you have a grasp of how your body is supposed to handle the food you eat, let's delve into what happens when things go wrong. Digestion problems grouped under the classification "nonulcer dyspepsia" are not caused by disease. Rather, they can be induced by nonstructural agents, such as certain foods and medications, as well as eating habits and stress. (Later in the chapter, we will take up digestion problems that are linked to such diseases as diabetes.) Nonulcer dyspepsia is the most frequent cause of dyspepsia symptoms and is diagnosed in one-quarter to one-third of all patients who undergo complete testing for dyspepsia. This diagnosis is made in a patient who has dyspepsia symptoms and in whom a standard diagnostic test (upper-GI endoscopy) reveals a normal esophagus, stomach, and upper small bowel.

Nonulcer dyspepsia may be due to several conditions, such as delayed emptying of the stomach, atypical (nonacid) reflux symptoms, or decreased ability of the stomach to distend normally to accommodate food. (See Figure 5.1.) It may also be due to increased sensitivity of the esophagus, stomach, or upper bowel to being stretched or distended; this is called *visceral hypersensitivity*. Yet another known cause of the condition is an infection in the stomach caused by a bacteria, e.g., *H. pylori*. This can be treated and improved with medication. Be sure to explore all diagnostic possibilities with your doctor.

One or two episodes of nonulcer dyspepsia symptoms—as long as they are not accompanied by any of the "red flag" symptoms listed in the following sidebar—are not particularly worrisome, especially if they subside on their own. In contrast, chronic dyspepsia, which may persist for weeks or months at a time, can make life miserable and disrupt your ability to provide healthy nourishment to your body. In the next sections, we will review some of the common causes of dyspepsia, as well as how to put your Four-Week Plan into gear for relief.

The main symptoms of nonulcer dyspepsia are of three types: refluxlike symptoms, ulcerlike symptoms, and slow-stomach symp-

Figure 5.1 **The Stomach's Role in Dyspepsia**

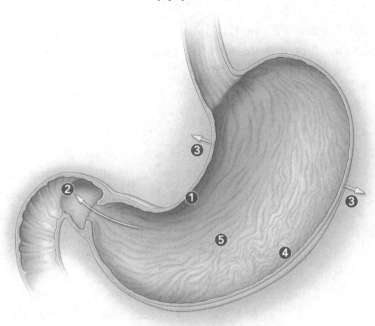

The stomach can be the source of several dyspepsia problems, as this diagram shows:

1. Erosion in the lining of the stomach, causing tiny ulcers
2. Altered or delayed emptying of food from the stomach into the duodenum (first part of the small bowel), causing bloating and abdominal cramps
3. Decreased ability of the stomach to expand normally with ingestion of a meal, i.e., decreased accommodation, causing dyspepsia
4. Food and medicine causes (see text)
5. Increased sensitivity of the lining of the stomach to its contents (visceral hyperalgesia).

toms. These symptoms may be related to what you eat, often in combination with structural problems with your digestive system. A fourth symptom, gas and bloating, is frequently related to what you eat and drink as well as to how you eat. Here is a symptom summary:

■ **Refluxlike symptoms.** Similar to the heartburn described in the preceding chapter, refluxlike symptoms are caused by food's reversing direction and heading back up into the esophagus.

WHEN TO SEEK HELP: DYSPEPSIA RED FLAGS

Please seek medical attention if your dyspepsia is accompanied by any of these symptoms:

- New onset of greater than ten pounds weight loss
- Blood in your stool
- Difficulty swallowing (*dysphagia*) or painful swallowing (*odynophagia*)
- Unpleasant or uncomfortable breathing (*dyspnea*)
- Unusual sweating (*diaphoresis*)
- Rapid or irregular heartbeat (*tachycardia*)
- New onset of persistent symptoms of dyspepsia after age forty-five
- Loss of appetite (*anorexia*)
- Persistent nausea and/or vomiting

- **Ulcerlike symptoms.** You feel a gnawing or burning pain in your stomach (upper part of the abdomen). You may also feel the pain in your back.

- **Slow-stomach symptoms.** These symptoms are related to digestion being slowed. The stomach is not emptying as quickly as it is getting filled; consequently, you feel bloated or distended, or you might feel a pressure in your stomach that makes you want to loosen your waistband. You may also feel uncomfortably full, as if you couldn't eat another bite (called *early satiety*). One of my patients described the feeling as, "I can chew, but I can't swallow!" Nausea and vomiting may be part of the picture as well.

- **Gas and bloating.** As you probably can attest, one of the most embarrassing and uncomfortable symptoms of dyspepsia is gas, which usually is accompanied by bloating. Practically speaking, gas is nothing to be embarrassed about: the body normally produces between half a quart and two quarts of gas every day! It needs to pass out of the body, so passing gas is a natural part of your digestion process. Problems come when too much gas is produced, causing bloating (uncomfortable fullness) and sometimes pain. Several foods and beverages known to cause gas are listed in the following section (see "Dyspepsia Food and Drink Culprits"). In addition to what you eat and drink, gas and bloating can be a product of the *way* you eat. Eating too quickly and swallowing air while you eat both contribute, as will be explained.

What Can Cause Dyspepsia?

The causes of dyspepsia fall into four main categories: foods, medications, eating habits, and structural problems or disease conditions. You have the most control over your choice of foods and your eating habits. You may have less control over the medications you are taking and certain disease conditions, while some structural problems can be treated medically or surgically corrected. In all circumstances, even those over which you have minimal control, you can usually take steps that will limit or reduce your symptoms.

Dyspepsia Food and Drink Culprits

Because dyspepsia encompasses such a wide variety of symptoms, many different foods can aggravate the condition. While everyone reacts differently, rich foods, fatty foods, and spicy foods are among the main culprits. Those french fries might be delicious, but when you eat fat, the bowel releases chemicals that slow down the stomach and keep it from emptying at its normal speed. I know it's a sacrifice to give up those rich, fatty, and fried foods, but those tempting treats may be behind your digestive discomfort.

Dairy and lactose-rich foods such as milk, cheese, ice cream, and yogurt can also leave you with dyspepsia symptoms. Lactose intolerance and lactose sensitivity are fairly common, so if you have a dairy-rich diet, it might be making your symptoms worse. If you think this is the case, be precise in recording what you are eating in your Food and Symptom Log, as well as associated symptoms such as gas, bloating, distension, and cramps. As you begin working on your Four-Week Plan, focus on how much dairy foods and fluids you consume. Remember to ask at restaurants whether your meal contains dairy—many dishes are cooked with butter or cream, even if it doesn't explicitly say that on the menu. As I've assured you before, people won't be insulted or irritated if you ask for a little more information; be polite, and explain that you're just trying to get a better idea of what you eat, because you have food sensitivities.

Remember those hard-to-digest diarrhea culprits from Chapter 2? Well, brassica vegetables and other high-fiber foods can also cause dyspepsia, simply because they are more difficult for your stomach and bowel to handle. Here are some highlights of those problematic foods:

- Beans of any variety
- Milk and milk products
- Fiber-rich salads
- Excess caffeine
- Colas and other carbonated beverages with a lot of sugar
- Sorbitol-containing foods, including peaches, pears, cherries, apples, apple juice, and pancake syrup

Recommended Alcohol Intake for Healthy Adults. It might be useful, as we run down dyspepsia food and drink culprits, to take note of the recommended amount of alcohol for healthy adults—that is, people without digestive or other health problems. If you find yourself exceeding these limits, I encourage you to have a discussion about your alcohol intake with your doctor.

One unit of alcohol is equal to ten grams, which is the amount in each of the following servings:

- One ounce of whiskey
- One twelve-ounce bottle of beer
- One four-ounce glass of wine

Recommended amounts for women are one unit per day or seven per week. For men, it is two units per day or fourteen per week. Many authorities advocate staying within these limits, and if you have dyspepsia, you should be even more careful about alcohol consumption.

Smoke Signals. Everything that you put into your mouth has the potential to affect your digestion. Although cigarettes aren't food, smoking has been shown to exacerbate symptoms of dyspepsia and other digestion-related problems.

Medications That Can Cause or Worsen Dyspepsia

In addition to the foods and drinks just specified, certain medications can have a significant effect on your dyspepsia symptoms. As with foods, any medications that slow your stomach down or interfere with proper digestive function are likely to make your symptoms worse. These include antihistamines such as Benadryl and Claritin, as well as antihypertensive medications such as calcium channel blockers. In addition, tricyclic antidepressants such as Zoloft, Paxil, and Cymbalta slow stomach emptying, as do diarrhea medications and pain medications. Examples of diarrhea medications that might intensify your symptoms are Imodium, Lomotil, and hyoscyamine. Similarly, numerous pain medications can affect stomach emptying and bowel transit, including codeine, morphine, Demerol, and Percocet. As you construct your Four-Week Plan, monitor your intake of any and all medications, but *do not stop taking prescription medications without talking to your doctor.*

The Way You Eat

Gaining control of your dyspepsia is not just a matter of changing *what* you eat and drink; it also calls for changing *how* you approach food and eating. Overeating compounds your symptoms, because you are filling your stomach faster than it can empty itself. In other words, overeating forces your stomach and bowel to work overtime. In addition to overeating, eating too quickly and swallowing air can put stress on your digestive system by causing bloating and gas. Think about how you approach mealtimes: Are you usually stressed out when you sit down to a meal? Is your mind on the bad day you had at work? Worst of all, are you gobbling down breakfast or lunch in the car?

Stress and similar emotions can make your dyspepsia symptoms much worse. As you start keeping your Food and Symptom Log, take some time to record your emotional state at mealtimes. The secret to relieving your symptoms may be as simple as relaxing a little, not only at mealtimes but also in your daily life! I'll talk about more ways to improve your eating habits later in the chapter.

Diseases and Conditions That Can Cause or Worsen Dyspepsia

Some diseases and conditions can team up with problem foods and medications to cause dyspepsia or make your symptoms more severe. If you know you have any of the conditions cited in this section, ask your doctor how it is affecting your digestive health. If you haven't been diagnosed with any of these conditions, it might still be a good idea to mention them to your doctor and ask if you've been tested.

First, endocrine and metabolic disorders, including diabetes and underactive thyroid, are among the most significant contributors to dyspepsia symptoms. Diabetes, in particular, is often accompanied by digestive symptoms. (Diabetes is covered in Chapter 7.) These symptoms usually fall into the category of dyspepsia, as diabetes can cause the stomach to empty more slowly. Why? Because when your blood sugar is higher than normal, it forces the stomach to slow down. Regulating your diabetes symptoms may help get your digestive problems under control. Talk to your doctor about the best way to do this.

Also, gallstones (pancreatic-biliary disease), *H. pylori gastritis* (an infection), functional GI disorders (such as IBS), and intestinal tract disorders that can cause diarrhea and constipation all prevent your digestive system from properly processing food and can produce or aggravate dyspepsia symptoms. You can ask your doctor to test you for these conditions if you are concerned.

▶Your Four-Week Plan for Dyspepsia

Since dyspepsia symptoms can be caused or worsened not only by food but also by your *eating habits*, pay careful attention to the *way* you are eating your meals as well what you are eating and drinking, and make it a practice to record these eating habits in your log. During the food-elimination week, focus particularly on these items:

- Rich, fatty, and spicy foods
- Milk and all other dairy products
- Carbonated beverages
- Alcohol
- Cigarettes

If you smoke, take steps to quit. I fully understand that making the decision to quit smoking is difficult, but you should be aware that lighting up might be affecting your digestive health, in addition to your general physical well-being. You don't have to do this alone! Talk to your doctor about strategies for quitting, and think seriously about whether you are now ready to take this giant step that could improve your life across the board. There are also many excellent smoking-cessation plans that your doctor can recommend.

While you are monitoring your food and drink intake, keep a close watch on any weight fluctuation. If you don't weigh yourself regularly, ask your doctor if you have recently gained or lost a significant amount of weight. There are two reasons for staying aware of your weight as you work toward a dyspepsia-free life. First, as the earlier "Red Flags" sidebar indicates, new onset of unexplained weight loss may be a sign of a serious medical condition that needs immediate treatment. Second, weight fluctuation can affect the severity of your dyspepsia symptoms. Gaining as little as ten pounds can make your symptoms much more troubling. Your doctor can give you suggestions and nutritional tips to help you achieve the healthiest weight, both for your symptoms and for your overall health and well-being. As a general guide, you should gain no more than three pounds between your morning weight and your weight at bedtime.

In addition to foods and drinks, take careful note of your medications, especially if you are currently taking any of the medications discussed in this chapter. Document your intake of and reaction to these medications, *but do not change medication intake at all without first talking to your doctor.*

Remember to Breathe!

During week two, expand your focus to encompass the *way* you are eating, which has particular relevance for dyspepsia. As you work to gain control of your digestive woes, take an inventory of how you approach meals and eating. Avoid overeating and eating too fast by putting your fork down between bites. Savor each bite of food, take the time to chew it properly, and don't rush to stuff the next bite into your mouth. Take a moment to breathe, inhale the aromas, and enjoy the flavor of what you are eating.

Another tried-and-true way to slow things down is by having a conversation. In Europe, for example, it is considered polite during a meal to put one's utensils down and ask accompanying family or friends about their day or engage them in a lively discussion. Perhaps that is why European meals sometimes last for hours! Even if you are eating alone, pause between bites to reflect on positive developments in your day and in your life. I do not recommend watching television while you eat, but listening to relaxing music can have a mellowing effect. You can also avoid overfilling your stomach by eating and drinking separately; a few sips of water are fine, but try not to fill your stomach with liquid in addition to a full meal.

I recommend that you plan to spend fifteen to twenty minutes eating a meal and that you swallow no fewer than sixty times per session. Don't cut all your meat or poultry into pieces before you eat it. Cutting one piece at a time and then swallowing it will help you to pace your eating. (Flip back to Chapter 1 for more details on healthy eating habits and portion control.) By avoiding eating rapidly, you will keep your consumption under control and not inhale your meals like a vacuum cleaner in five minutes flat.

Helpful Foods

During weeks three and four, as you eliminate troublesome foods and begin to add back foods that help, here are some suggested additions that can aid in relieving dyspepsia symptoms: white rice, white bread, chicken, fish, turkey, bananas, cooked green beans and peas, simple salads (iceberg lettuce and tomato), and homemade vegetable or chicken soups. If you try these, precisely note your reactions in your log.

Transform What You Drink

If you are accustomed to downing a carbonated beverage with every meal, this habit may be contributing to your dyspepsia and gas problem. As you undertake maintenance of your Food and Symptom Log, remember that drinks count too! Be cognizant of how many carbonated beverages and other gas-causing foods you consume each day. It can become second nature to order a soda at a restaurant or to grab one out of the fridge. Avoid this reflex by directing your attention to your food, rather than automatically chugging a soda with every meal. Think about how much more you'll enjoy your meal without that sugary, carbonated drink spoiling the flavor. In the grocery, try to avoid buying carbonated drinks, so that you won't have them on hand at home.

If you're craving something other than water, try making your own fresh vegetable or fruit juice, without adding sugar. (Always pay attention to the amount of sugar in your beverages.) Don't overdo the juices, though; too much fruit juice can aggravate your symptoms as well. You may want to give the flavored, noncarbonated waters a whirl or, better yet, use fresh fruit to flavor a normal glass of water. Go beyond a slice of lemon and be adventurous! Try freezing raspberries or blueberries in ice cubes, and give that glass of water some color and flavor. Use your favorite fruits to make delicious, original beverages that don't have digestive consequences.

Alcohol Watch

While we're talking about beverages, it is important to know that alcohol may also be causing some of your symptoms. Alcohol consumption can interfere with proper digestive function, so you should monitor your alcohol intake carefully as you work on your Four-Week Plan. Compounding the alcohol problem are cocktails that contain carbonated or sugary mixers such as soda, syrup, or fruit juice, which can exacerbate your dyspepsia. It's easy to consume a large quantity of these mixers even if you have only a couple of drinks.

If you tend to drink alcohol every day, try changing those after-work drink dates to coffee or tea dates during your food-elimination week. Explain to your friends that you're trying to make yourself healthier. Perhaps they will follow your example, and you might discover a delicious new nonalcoholic beverage! In all likelihood, you won't have to completely give up drinking alcohol permanently, but make sure you test and understand its effect on you during your Four-Week Plan. (See the alcohol intake recommendations earlier in the chapter.)

Dyspepsia Bottom Line

The chief message that the uncomfortable indigestion symptoms of dyspepsia are sending is that you are not only *what* you eat but also *how* you eat. Your Four-Week Plan will help you work with your doctor to take control of your diet, while at home you work on creating relaxing and healthy mealtimes. Even after you have completed your Four-Week Plan, continue those relaxing mealtime habits you have developed.

Staying positive, relaxed, and stress free while you eat works wonders. Whatever is going on in your life, look on mealtimes as a welcome escape from the stress you might experience throughout the rest of the day. Eschew conversations about subjects that elicit tension or stress, and create a peaceful atmosphere conducive to simply savoring your food. If you are alone, you might want to read an interesting book or ponder the positive aspects of your life. Enjoy your meal on an attractive plate, and sip your water from a beautiful glass. Finish your meal with a relaxing cup of (decaffeinated or herbal) tea, and try to draw that peaceful feeling into the next stage of your day.

DIGESTIVE DETECTIVE WORK

A young woman, Marian W., in my office looked more as if she should be running around on a soccer field than slumped in a hospital chair. She was a twenty-three-year-old college student, but her digestive problems were interrupting every part of her life. For the previous six weeks, she had been experiencing bloating, distension of her abdomen, nausea, and the inability to eat a normal-size meal. "I get full halfway through the meal and have to stop eating," she said, "and this is not like me at all. I used to love food!" Because of this state of affairs, she had lost eight pounds in just a few weeks. "Losing weight is great," she said with a sigh, "but this is not the way I'd like to do it."

This young woman's condition resembled a form of dyspepsia: recurrent upper-abdominal discomfort that can include some combination of refluxlike symptoms, ulcerlike symptoms, and slow-stomach symptoms. In her case, the nausea, bloating, and feeling of fullness suggested the third condition, which is also called *gastroparesis*. Before making a definitive diagnosis, however, I needed to learn more.

A few weeks previously, she had gone to another physician, who had performed an endoscopic examination, in which a tube is inserted through the mouth that allows the doctor to see inside the stomach. The test results were normal, revealing no structural or mechanical reason for her symptoms. The doctor had advised her to try over-the-counter medicines such as Prilosec (omeprazole) or Zantac (ranitidine), but nothing had helped.

Clearly, some digestive detective work was needed. I took a more detailed medical history and discovered that eight weeks earlier, just before her symptoms started, she had had an upper-respiratory infection with coughing, a sore throat, and muscle aches, as well as a low-grade fever. As you have read in this chapter, viral infections such as this may induce the stomach to empty more slowly than normal, giving way to the symptoms of slow-stomach dyspepsia. If the stomach does not empty as quickly as it is getting filled, you feel bloated or distended, or you might feel a pressure in your stomach that makes you want to loosen your belt. You may also feel uncomfortably full, as if you can't eat another morsel (*early satiety*).

To find out if slow stomach emptying was causing my patient's problems, I had her undergo a special nuclear medicine study in which she ate a meal with eggs, along with tracer doses of a nuclear material that allows the rate of stomach emptying to be measured. Normally, half the test meal should be out of the stomach within sixty minutes and on its way to the bowel to be eliminated. In her case, most of the meal was still in her stomach after three hours! The onset of her symptoms six to eight weeks after her viral infection—and in the presence of a normal endoscopic examination of her stomach—strongly suggested that her dyspepsia had been triggered by the illness and could be treated effectively.

A medication designed to speed up stomach emptying began to give her relief from her symptoms within two weeks, and she was able to tolerate four or five small meals a day without bloating, distension, or nausea. A month after that, she was back to her normal eating habits and able to decrease the use of the medication. At a six-month follow-up, she was off the medication. "I feel wonderful," she reported to me during her final check-up. "Now, can you do anything to improve college cafeteria food?"

Chapter 6

Celiac Sprue

T he smell of fresh-baked bread is a comforting, irresistible aroma for most people. For you, alas, tantalizing bites of bread might be synonymous with a bloated stomach, abdominal pain, or diarrhea. These symptoms, along with many others, could indicate that you have celiac sprue. The terms *celiac disease* and *sprue* are interchangeable, and the term used in this chapter will be *celiac sprue*. This is a surprisingly common genetic condition in which people who are predisposed by a genetic abnormality cannot digest gluten normally.

Gluten is a protein that is present in wheat, rye, barley, and malt. It is also often used as a coating for some vitamins and medicines and as a stabilizer in processed foods and bottled sauces. When people with celiac sprue eat foods containing gluten, the breakdown products during digestion both alter the lining of the small bowel and trigger an immune response that causes further damage. It is considered an "autoimmune" disorder, because the body is actually stimulated to attack a part of itself—in this case, the lining of the small intestine.

▶The Damage of Celiac Sprue

The small intestine, as mentioned in the preceding chapter, is normally lined with tiny, hairlike projections called *villi*. As the

Figure 6.1 **The Damaging Effects of Gluten**

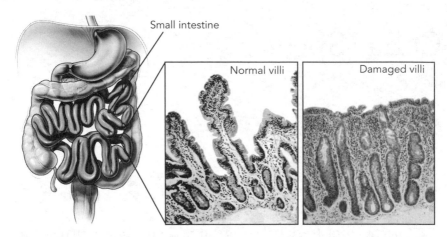

In celiac sprue, gluten (found in many foods) triggers the body to "attack" and damage nutrient-absorbing villi in the small intestine, interfering with the capacity to transfer nutrients from the intestine into the bloodstream. The box at right shows damaged villi, compared with healthy villi to the left.

partially digested food you eat passes through the intestine, these villi pull the nutrients out of the food and into your bloodstream. If you have celiac sprue, however, any gluten you eat triggers your body's immune system to attack and damage these villi. (See Figure 6.1.) With damaged villi, your body cannot absorb nutrients normally from your food, no matter how nutritious it is or how much you eat.

In this chapter, we explore celiac sprue causes, symptoms, and treatments. I'm pleased to report that there is much you can do, by controlling your diet, to reduce or eliminate your symptoms. This will be the basis for your Four-Week Plan for celiac sprue.

▶Symptoms of Celiac Sprue

This is a complex disease, with a range of possible symptoms. Not everyone has every symptom, because people's gluten intolerance manifests in individual ways. The "classic" form of the disease develops in childhood and is controlled by adhering to a permanent gluten-free diet. The "latent" form of the disease has two types: (1) a diagnosis in childhood, management with a gluten-free diet, and remaining symptom free even after resuming a normal diet; and (2) development later in life, while on a normal diet. If you suspect that you have celiac sprue after reading about the following symptoms, see your doctor for a diagnosis. The symptoms can be grouped by type:

- **Abdominal symptoms.** The abdominal symptoms, as first mentioned in Chapter 2, are often confused with irritable bowel. They include bloating, gas, constipation, diarrhea, recurring stomach pain, and stool that is foul smelling, fatty, and pale.

- **Muscle and bone symptoms.** These can manifest as muscle cramps, bone or joint pain, tingling or numbness in the legs, osteoporosis (weak, brittle bones prone to breaking), and osteopenia (a preosteoporosis condition).

- **Body symptoms.** Sufferers may experience anemia, fatigue, weight loss or gain, swelling of the feet and legs, failure to thrive in infants, itchy skin rash (called *dermatitis herpetiformis*), delayed growth in children, tooth discoloration or loss of enamel, and mouth sores (called *aphthous ulcers*).

- **Women's symptoms.** Women with celiac sprue are at risk for missed menstrual periods, infertility, and recurrent miscarriages.

Several of these symptoms are associated with malnutrition. For example, anemia indicates poor absorption of dietary iron; osteoporosis indicates poor calcium absorption; and missed menstrual periods sometimes occur with severe weight loss. This happens because the body is not properly absorbing the nutrients from food.

Celiac Sprue-Related Complications

Even if you have no symptoms, you still might have the disease and can be at risk for the complications, including malnutrition and its consequences: in particular, anemia and osteoporosis. In addition to malnutrition, damage to the small intestine creates an increased risk for lymphoma and adenocarcinoma, cancers that develop in the small intestine. Some people with celiac disease are also shorter than the average height. This is because the disease interferes with the absorption of nutrients from food during the critical early growth years of childhood.

Because celiac sprue is an autoimmune disease—meaning that one part of the body "attacks" another part, mistaking it for a "foreign enemy invader"—people with celiac disease may also be at risk for other autoimmune diseases. These include rheumatoid arthritis, type 1 diabetes, thyroid disease, and lupus. This is why early diagnosis is so important.

Diagnosing Celiac Sprue

Celiac sprue is often either *mis*diagnosed or *under*diagnosed. This is because the symptoms can be confused with those of other maladies, including irritable bowel syndrome, anemia that is thought to be caused by the loss of menstrual blood, diverticulitis, intestinal infections, and chronic fatigue syndrome.

Fortunately, thanks to recent scientific advances, the diagnosis has become much easier. People with celiac sprue have been shown to have higher-than-normal levels of certain autoantibodies in their blood. An antibody is like a soldier in the army of the immune system, called out to protect the body from threats that the immune system identifies as "foreign," or dangerous, such as viruses and bacteria. An autoantibody is an antibody that reacts against the body's own molecules or tissues, raining the equivalent of "friendly fire" on parts of the body that are not dangerous at all

RED FLAGS: WHEN TO SEEK MEDICAL ATTENTION FOR CELIAC SPRUE

Even if you are under a doctor's care, the following symptoms should prompt you to seek medical attention:

- Diarrhea that persists for more than two months
- Weight loss of more than eight pounds over a six-month period
- Consistent symptoms after eating gluten-containing foods
- Weakness and tiring easily
- Unexplained change in menstrual cycle
- Easy bruising
- Getting up at night to urinate
- Bone pain
- Numbness and tingling in the arms and legs

and causing serious damage. This is what happens in type 1 diabetes, for example, when the body attacks its own insulin-producing cells of the pancreas, and in multiple sclerosis, when the body attacks its own protective coverings of nerves.

The same phenomenon of an immune system that has "run amok" results in damage to the villi of the small intestine. The promising development in this regard is that now doctors are able to test your blood to determine if you have these celiac sprue–related autoantibodies. Your doctor will want to measure your levels of the following substances:

- Immunoglobulin A (IgA)
- Tissue transglutaminase antibodies (tTGA)
- IgA anti-endomysial antibodies (AEA)

It is necessary that you continue to eat foods with gluten before your test, as you may test falsely negative after four to six weeks on a gluten-free diet, because the level of these antibodies will drop. If the test and your symptoms suggest that you have celiac sprue, your doctor will then perform a biopsy of your small intestine. This is a relatively easy endoscopic procedure in which a small, thin tube is inserted down through your mouth into the small intestine. The doctor will then examine the sample that comes back through the tube to see if the intestine lining is altered and lacks normal villi to properly absorb the nutrients from the food you eat.

Even if you don't receive the diagnosis of celiac sprue, however, you might have a gluten sensitivity. This condition, which is common among people who consume too much gluten, causes digestion problems similar to those of dyspepsia (described in Chapter 5). While the treatment for celiac sprue is complete elimination of gluten from the diet, you might not have to go to that extreme if all you have is a gluten sensitivity, without the destructive effects of the autoantibodies on the lining of your small intestine.

Depending on what you have, the Four-Week Plan will vary. If you have a confirmed diagnosis of celiac sprue through blood tests and small-bowel biopsy, you must not add back any gluten-containing foods during week four. Instead, you need to completely and permanently revamp your diet, and I will give you some suggestions of how to do this. If, instead, you have only a gluten sensitivity, there may be foods—such as flours other than wheat—that you will be able to add back into your diet, depending on your reactions to them during week three.

▶Your Four-Week Plan for Celiac Sprue

While your disease may be more complicated than other problems outlined in this book, your solution is going to be relatively straightforward. If you have been diagnosed with celiac sprue, we already know that gluten is your problem. This means that you can forgo much of the experimental "ABAB" period during weeks three and four. Instead, you can begin to explore your new food guidelines and learn about the hidden sources of gluten.

The only treatment for celiac sprue is to follow a gluten-free diet. This demands constant attentiveness, since gluten is hidden in many foods that you would probably not suspect, including additives such as modified food starch, preservatives, and stabilizers. Because some vitamins and medications also contain gluten, as do many bottled sauces and condiments, it is incumbent on you to scrutinize labels and to seek guidance from a registered dietitian or nutritionist regarding your food and supplement choices. Use Table 6.1 and the companion notes in Tables 6.2, 6.3, and 6.4 as your reference lists of safe, questionable, and forbidden foods, and do not neglect to alert restaurant staff or anyone else who prepares food for you of your gluten intolerance.

As a first step, train your sights on constructing your diet with plain meat, poultry, fish, rice, and fresh fruits and vegetables. As you bid good-bye to forbidden foods—such as wheat, rye, barley, triticale, spelt, bulgur, and other gluten-rich flours—you make way for some new and versatile gluten-free flours, including teff, amaranth, arrowroot, buckwheat, corn, millet, tapioca, potato, and bean flours. There are now many celiac websites offering a multitude of recipes, as well as "safe" flours and other food products for sale. Some good places to begin online are celiacsprue.org and csa celiacs.org/celiac_defined.php.

You also might want to join a celiac support group, since making a wide-ranging change to your eating habits on your own can be daunting. Many people with celiac invest in a bread machine and make delicious, gluten-free breads at home. So, that aroma of freshly baked bread, muffins, or pancakes can still tantalize you— but safely!

What About Gluten Sensitivity?

If your Food and Symptom Log shows a sensitivity to gluten—for example, you respond with bloating, gas, congestion, or diarrhea— and your doctor has ruled out celiac sprue, you should take a more conventional approach to your Four-Week Plan. By week three, you should have a fairly good idea of the foods that are causing your problems. During week three, carefully record your symptoms after eating and then eliminating all of these variations. During week four, add one type of product back at a time, and observe

Table 6.1 Gluten-Free Diet by Food Groups

Food Category	Foods Allowed (See Table 6.2)	Foods to Question (See Table 6.3)	Foods to Avoid (See Table 6.4)
Milk and Dairy	Milk, cream, most ice cream, buttermilk, plain yogurt, cheese, cream cheese, processed cheese, processed cheese foods, cottage cheese	Flavored yogurt, frozen yogurt, cheese sauces, cheese spreads, seasoned (flavored) shredded cheese	Malted milk, ice cream made with ingredients not allowed
Grains and Starches	**Breads, Baked Products, and Other Items:** Items made with amaranth, arrowroot, buckwheat, corn bran, corn flour, cornmeal, cornstarch, flax, legume flours (bean, garbanzo [chickpea], garfava, lentil, pea), mesquite flour, millet, Montina flour (Indian rice grass), nut flours (almond, chestnut, hazelnut), potato flour, potato starch, pure uncontaminated oat products (oat flour, oat groats, oatmeal), quinoa, rice bran, rice flours (brown, glutinous, sweet, white), rice polish, sago, sorghum flour, soy flour, sweet potato flour, tapioca (cassava, manioc), taro, and teff

Cereals—Hot: Puffed amaranth, cornmeal, cream of buckwheat, cream of rice (brown, white), hominy grits, pure uncontaminated oatmeal, quinoa | Items made with buckwheat flour

Rice flakes, soy flakes, soy grits, and soy and rice pablum | Items made with wheat bran, wheat farina, wheat flour, wheat germ, wheat-based semolina, wheat starch,* durum flour, gluten flour, graham flour, atta, bulgur, einkorn, emmer, farro, kamut, spelt, barley, rye, and triticale, and commercial oat products (oat bran, oat flour, oat groats, oatmeal)

Cereals made from wheat, rye, triticale, barley, and commercial oats |

	Cereals—Cold: Puffed amaranth, buckwheat, corn, millet, and rice, rice crisps and corn flakes (with no barley malt extract or barley malt flavoring), rice flakes, soy cereals	Rice and corn cereals	Cereals made with added barley malt extract or barley malt flavoring
	Pastas: Macaroni, spaghetti, and noodles made from beans, corn, lentils, peas, potatoes, quinoa, rice, soy, and wild rice	Buckwheat pasta	Pastas made from wheat, wheat starch, and other ingredients not allowed, such as orzo
	Rice: Plain (basmati, brown, jasmine, white, wild)	Seasoned (flavored) rice mixes	
	Miscellaneous: Corn tacos, corn tortillas, rice tortillas		Wheat flour tacos and tortillas, matzo, matzo meal, matzo balls, couscous, tabbouleh
	Plain rice crackers, rice cakes, and corn cakes	Multigrain and flavored rice crackers, rice cakes, and corn cakes	
	Gluten-free communion wafers	Low-gluten communion wafers	Regular communion wafers
Meats and Alternatives	**Meat, Fish, and Poultry:** Plain (fresh and frozen)	Deli and luncheon meats (bologna, salami), wieners, frankfurters, sausages, pâté, meat and sandwich spreads, frozen burgers (meat, fish, chicken), meat loaf, ham (ready to cook), dried meats such as beef jerky, seasoned (flavored) fish in pouches, imitation fish products such as surimi, meat substitutes, meat product extenders	Canned fish in vegetable broth containing hydrolyzed wheat protein; frozen turkey basted or injected with hydrolyzed wheat protein; frozen and fresh turkey with bread stuffing; frozen chicken breasts containing chicken broth (made with ingredients not allowed); meat, poultry, and fish breaded in ingredients not allowed

(continued)

Table 6.1 Gluten-Free Diet by Food Groups *(continued)*

Food Category	Foods Allowed (See Table 6.2)	Foods to Question (See Table 6.3)	Foods to Avoid (See Table 6.4)
	Eggs: Fresh, liquid, dried, and powdered	Flavored egg products (liquid and frozen)	
	Others: Dried beans (black, garbanzo [also known as chickpea, besan, channa, or gram], kidney, navy, pinto, soy, white), dried peas, lentils	Baked beans	
	Plain nuts and seeds (chia, flax, sesame, pumpkin, sunflower), and nut and seed butters (almond, peanut, sesame)	Seasoned and dry-roasted nuts, seasoned pumpkin and sunflower seeds	
	Plain tofu	Flavored tofu, tempeh, miso	Fu, seitan
Fruits and Vegetables	**Fruits:** Fresh, frozen, and canned fruits and juices	Dates, fruits with sauces	
	Vegetables: Fresh, frozen, and canned vegetables and juices	Vegetables with sauces, french-fried potatoes cooked in oil also used for gluten-containing products	Scalloped potatoes (containing wheat flour), battered deep-fried vegetables
Soups	Gluten-free bouillon cubes and homemade broth, cream soups, and stocks made with allowed ingredients	Canned soups, dried soup mixes, soup bases, bouillon cubes	Soups made with ingredients not allowed, bouillon cubes containing hydrolyzed wheat protein

	Foods Allowed		Foods Not Allowed
Fats	Butter, margarine, lard, shortening, vegetable oils, salad dressings made with allowed ingredients	Salad dressings, suet, cooking sprays	Salad dressings made with ingredients not allowed
Desserts	Ice cream, sherbet, whipped toppings, whipping cream, milk puddings, custard, gelatin desserts, cakes, cookies, pies, and pastries made with allowed ingredients	Cake icings and frostings	Bread pudding, ice cream made with ingredients not allowed such as cookie crumbs, and cakes, cookies, muffins, pies, and pastries made with ingredients not allowed
	Gluten-free ice cream cones, wafers, and waffles		Ice cream cones, wafers, and waffles made with ingredients not allowed
Others	**Sweets:** Honey, jam, jelly, marmalade, corn syrup, maple syrup, molasses, sugar (brown and white), icing sugar (confectioners')	Honey powder	
	Gluten-free licorice, marshmallows	Hard candies, Smarties, chocolates, chocolate bars	Licorice and other candies made with ingredients not allowed
	Snack Foods: Plain popcorn, nuts, soy nuts, potato chips, taco (corn) chips	Seasoned (flavored) potato chips, taco (corn) chips, nuts, soy nuts	Potato chips made with ingredients not allowed
	Gluten-free pizza		Pizza made with ingredients not allowed
	Beverages: Tea, instant and ground coffee (regular and decaffeinated), cocoa, soft drinks	Flavored and herbal teas, flavored coffees, coffee substitutes, hot chocolate mixes	Cereal- and malt-based beverages such as Ovaltine (chocolate malt and malt flavor) and Postum

(continued)

Table 6.1 Gluten-Free Diet by Food Groups *(continued)*

Food Category	Foods Allowed (See Table 6.2)	Foods to Question (See Table 6.3)	Foods to Avoid (See Table 6.4)
	Distilled alcoholic beverages (bourbon, gin, rum, rye whiskey, Scotch whisky, vodka, liqueurs), wine	Flavored alcoholic beverages (coolers, ciders, Caesar vodka beverage)	
	Gluten-free beer, ale, and lager		Beer, ale, and lager derived from barley
	Most nondairy beverages made from nuts, potatoes, rice, and soy		Nondairy beverages (nut, potato, rice, soy) made with barley malt extract, barley malt flavoring, and oats
	Condiments and Sauces: Ketchup, relish, plain prepared mustard, pure mustard flour, herbs, spices, salt, pepper, olives, plain pickles, tomato paste, vinegars (apple or cider, balsamic, distilled white, grape or wine, rice, spirit), gluten-free soy sauce, gluten-free teriyaki sauce, other sauces and gravies made with allowed ingredients	Specialty prepared mustards, prepared mustard flour, mustard pickles, Worcestershire sauce, curry paste	Malt vinegar, soy sauce (made from wheat), teriyaki sauce (made with soy sauce containing wheat), other sauces and gravies made with wheat flour or hydrolyzed wheat protein

	Baking powder	Brewer's yeast
Miscellaneous: Plain cocoa, pure baking chocolate, carob chips and powder, chocolate chips, baking soda, cream of tartar, coconut, monosodium glutamate (MSG), vanilla, pure vanilla extract, artificial (synthetic, imitation) vanilla extract, vanillin, yeast (active dry, autolyzed, baker's, nutritional, torula), xanthan gum, guar gum		

Courtesy of Shelley Case, RD, author of *Gluten-Free Diet: A Comprehensive Resource Guide*; Medical Advisory Board Member–Celiac Disease Foundation; Gluten Intolerance Group; and Canadian Celiac Association

*Imported foods labeled "gluten-free" made with wheat starch.

Table 6.2 Notes for Table 6.1 on Foods Allowed

Food Category	Food Products	Notes
Grains and Starches	Garfava flour	A specialty flour made from garbanzo beans (chickpeas) and fava beans, developed by Authentic Foods.
	Mesquite flour	Made from the ground pods of the mesquite tree.
	Montina flour	Made from Indian rice grass.
	Quinoa	A small seed of a South American plant that can be cooked and eaten whole or ground into flour or flakes.
	Glutinous rice flour	Also known as sweet, sticky, or sushi rice flour. Made from a sticky short-grain rice that is higher in starch than brown or white rice. Does not contain any gluten.
	Sago	An edible starch derived from the pith of the stems of a certain variety of palm trees. Usually ground into a powder and used as a thickener or dense flour.
	Tapioca (cassava, manioc, yucca)	A tropical plant that produces a starchy edible root that is peeled and can be boiled, baked, or fried. The peeled root can also be dried and washed with water to extract the starch (known as tapioca starch), which can be used to make baked products and tapioca pearls.
	Taro (dasheen, eddo)	A tropical plant harvested for its large, starchy tubers, which are consumed as a cooked vegetable or made into breads, puddings, or poi (a Polynesian dish).
	Teff	A tiny seed of a grass native to Ethiopia that can be cooked and eaten whole or ground into flour.
	Hominy grits (corn grits)	Coarsely or finely ground corn kernels that are cooked and eaten as a hot breakfast cereal or side dish.
	Gluten-free communion wafers	No-gluten hosts made from soy and rice flour by Ener-G Foods. These hosts are allowed by most major denominations except the Catholic Church.

Meats and Alternatives	Chia	An oilseed of the ancient plant species *Salvia hispanica L.* It belongs to the mint family and is grown in Central and South America. Available in a natural brown and white seed, sold as chia; a pure white variety is sold under the brand Salba. It is high in omega-3 fatty acids and fiber. The seed should be ground to get the maximum benefit of all the nutritional components.
Others	Distilled alcoholic beverages	Rye whiskey, Scotch whisky, gin, vodka, and bourbon are distilled from a mash of fermented grains. Although they are derived from a gluten-containing grain, the distillation process removes the gluten from the purified final product. Rum (distilled from sugarcane) and brandy (distilled from wine) are also gluten free. Liqueurs (also known as cordials) are made from an infusion of a distilled alcoholic beverage and flavoring agents such as nuts, fruits, seeds, and cream.
	Gluten-free beer, ale, and lager	Can be made from fermented rice, buckwheat, millet, and/or sorghum.
	Plain prepared mustard	Made from distilled vinegar, water, mustard seed, salt, spices, and flavors.
	Pure mustard flour	A powder made from pure ground mustard seed.
	Vinegars	Produced from various ingredients: balsamic (grapes), cider (apples), rice (rice wine), white distilled (corn, wheat, or both), wine (red wine). All of these vinegars are gluten free (including distilled white derived from wheat, as the distillation process removes the gluten from the final purified product), except for malt vinegar.
	Vanilla	Pure vanilla and pure vanilla extract are derived from the vanilla bean pods of a climbing orchid grown in tropical locations. The vanilla beans are chopped, soaked in alcohol and water, aged, and then filtered. Must contain at least 35% ethyl alcohol by volume. The pure vanilla is bottled; the pure extract can be mixed with sugar and a stabilizer and then bottled.

(continued)

Table 6.2 Notes for Table 6.1 on Foods Allowed (*continued*)

Food Category	Food Products	Notes
	Natural vanilla flavor	Derived from vanilla beans but contains less than 35% ethyl alcohol. May also contain sugar and a stabilizer.
	Artificial (synthetic, imitation) vanilla extract, vanillin	Made from a by-product of the pulp and paper industry or a coal-tar derivative that is chemically treated to mimic the flavor of vanilla. Also contains alcohol, water, color, and a stabilizer.
	Autolyzed yeast and autolyzed yeast extract	A special process causes yeast to be broken down by its own enzymes, resulting in the production of various compounds that can be used as flavoring agents. Autolyzed yeast is almost always derived from baker's yeast.
	Baker's yeast	A type of yeast grown on sugar beet molasses. It is available as active dry yeast granules (sold in packets or jars) or compressed yeast (also known as wet yeast, cake yeast, or fresh yeast), which must be refrigerated.
	Nutritional yeast	A specific strain of an inactive form of baker's yeast that is grown on a mixture of sugar beet molasses and then fermented, washed, pasteurized, and dried at high temperatures. Used as a dietary supplement, it contains protein, fiber, vitamins, and minerals. Available in pills, flakes, and powder.
	Torula yeast	A yeast grown on wood sugars (a by-product of the pulp and paper industry). Used as a flavoring agent, it has a hickory smoke characteristic.
	Xanthan gum	This powder, produced from the fermentation of corn sugar, is used to thicken sauces and salad dressings and in gluten-free baked products to improve the structure and texture.
	Guar gum	A gum extracted from the seed of an East Indian plant. Available as a powder that is used as a thickener and stabilizer. Can be substituted for xanthan gum in gluten-free baked products. It is high in fiber and may have a laxative effect if consumed in large amounts.

Courtesy of Shelley Case, RD, author of *Gluten-Free Diet: A Comprehensive Resource Guide*; Medical Advisory Board Member—Celiac Disease Foundation; Gluten Intolerance Group; and Canadian Celiac Association

Table 6.3 Notes for Table 6.1 on Foods to Question

Food Category	Food Products	Notes
Milk and Dairy	Flavored yogurt, frozen yogurt	May contain granola, cookie crumbs, or wheat bran.
	Cheese sauces such as nacho, cheese spreads, seasoned (flavored) shredded cheese	May be thickened with wheat flour or wheat starch. Seasonings may contain hydrolyzed wheat protein, wheat flour, or wheat starch.
Grains and Starches	Buckwheat flour	Pure buckwheat flour is gluten free; however, some buckwheat flour may be mixed with wheat flour.
	Rice and corn cereals	May contain barley malt, barley malt extract, or barley malt flavoring.
	Buckwheat pasta	Also called Japanese soba noodles. Some soba pasta contains pure buckwheat flour, which is gluten free, but others may also contain wheat flour.
	Seasoned (flavored) rice mixes	Seasonings may contain hydrolyzed wheat protein, wheat flour, or wheat starch or have added soy sauce (made from wheat).
	Multigrain and flavored rice crackers, rice cakes, and corn cakes	Multigrain products may contain barley and/or oats. Some contain soy sauce (made from wheat) and/or seasonings with hydrolyzed wheat protein, wheat flour, or wheat starch.

(continued)

Table 6.3 Notes for Table 6.1 on Foods to Question *(continued)*

Food Category	Food Products	Notes
	Low-gluten communion wafers	The Catholic Canon Law, code 924.2, requires the presence of some wheat in communion wafers and will not accept the gluten-free hosts made with other grains. A very low-gluten host made with a small amount of specially processed wheat starch is available from the Benedictine Sisters of Perpetual Hope. The level of gluten in these hosts is extremely small (less than 37 micrograms, or 0.037 milligram per wafer). The Italian Celiac Association's scientific committee approved the use of the low-gluten host. Many health professionals endorse the use of this host. Some recommend consuming only a fourth of a wafer per week. The decision of whether to use this host should be discussed with your health professional. The hosts can be purchased by calling (800) 223-2772, e-mailing altarbreads@benedictinesisters.org, or writing to Benedictine Sisters Altar Bread Department, 31970 State Highway P, Clyde, MO 64432. More information for Catholics with celiac disease can be found at catholicceliacs.org.
Meats and Alternatives	Deli and luncheon meats, wieners, sausages, dried meats	May contain fillers made from wheat. Seasonings may contain hydrolyzed wheat protein, wheat flour, or wheat starch.
	Meat and sandwich spreads	Products such as pâté may contain wheat flour or seasonings with hydrolyzed wheat protein, wheat flour, or wheat starch.
	Frozen burgers (meat, fish, chicken), meat loaf	May contain fillers (wheat flour, wheat starch, bread crumbs). Seasonings may contain hydrolyzed wheat protein, wheat flour, or wheat starch.
	Ham (ready to cook)	Glaze may contain hydrolyzed wheat protein, wheat flour, or wheat starch.
	Seasoned (flavored) fish in pouches	May contain wheat or barley.

	Imitation fish products such as surimi	Imitation crab and other seafood sticks may contain fillers such as wheat starch.
	Meat substitutes (vegetarian burgers, sausages, roasts, nuggets, textured vegetable protein)	Often contain hydrolyzed wheat protein, wheat gluten, wheat starch, or barley malt.
	Flavored egg products (frozen and liquid)	May contain hydrolyzed wheat protein.
	Baked beans	Some are thickened with wheat flour.
	Seasoned and dry-roasted nuts, seasoned pumpkin and sunflower seeds	May contain hydrolyzed wheat protein, wheat flour, or wheat starch.
	Flavored tofu	May contain soy sauce (made from wheat) or other seasonings with hydrolyzed wheat protein, wheat flour, or wheat starch.
	Tempeh	A meat substitute made from fermented soybeans and millet or rice. Often seasoned with soy sauce (made from wheat).
	Miso	A condiment used in Asian cooking made from fermented soybeans and/or barley, wheat, or rice. Wheat and barley are the most common grains used.
Fruits and Vegetables	Dates	Chopped, diced, and extruded dates are packaged with oat flour, dextrose, or rice flour. Oat flour and dextrose are the most common sources used.
	French-fried potatoes	Often cooked in the same oil as gluten-containing foods such as breaded fish and chicken fingers, resulting in cross-contamination.

(continued)

Table 6.3 Notes for Table 6.1 on Foods to Question (continued)

Food Category	Food Products	Notes
Soups	Canned soups, dried soup mixes, soup bases, bouillon cubes	May contain noodles or barley. Cream soups are often thickened with wheat flour. Seasonings may contain hydrolyzed wheat protein, wheat flour, or wheat starch.
Fats	Salad dressings	May contain wheat flour, malt vinegar, or soy sauce (made from wheat). Seasonings may contain hydrolyzed wheat protein, wheat flour, or wheat starch.
	Suet	The hard fat around the loins and kidneys of beef and sheep. Flour may be added to packaged suet. Suet can be used to make mincemeat, steamed Christmas pudding, and haggis (a traditional Scottish dish).
	Cooking sprays	May contain wheat flour or wheat starch.
Desserts	Cake icing and frostings	May contain wheat flour or wheat starch.
Others	Honey powder	This commercial powder is used in glazes, seasoning mixes, dry mixes, and sauces. May contain wheat flour or wheat starch.
	Hard candies and chocolates	May contain barley malt flavoring and/or wheat flour.
	Smarties	A Canadian product that contains wheat flour.
	Chocolate bars	May contain wheat flour or barley malt flavoring.
	Seasoned (flavored) potato chips, taco (corn) chips, nuts, soy nuts	Some potato chips contain wheat starch. Seasoning mixes may contain hydrolyzed wheat protein, wheat flour, or wheat starch.

Flavored and herbal teas, flavored coffees	May contain barley malt flavoring. Some specialty coffees may be prepared with a chocolate chip–like product that contains cookie crumbs.
Coffee substitutes	Roasted chicory is the most common coffee substitute and is gluten free. Other coffee substitutes are derived from wheat, rye, barley, and/or malted barley.
Hot chocolate mixes	May contain barley malt or wheat starch.
Flavored alcoholic beverages	May contain barley malt.
Specialty prepared mustards	Some brands contain wheat flour.
Prepared mustard flour	Made from ground mustard seed, sugar, salt, and spices, which are gluten free; however, some brands also contain wheat flour.
Mustard pickles	May contain wheat flour and/or malt vinegar.
Worcestershire sauce	May contain malt vinegar.
Curry paste	Made from the pulp of the tamarind pod and a variety of spices. Some curry pastes may also contain wheat flour or wheat starch.
Baking powder	Most brands contain cornstarch, which is gluten free; however, some brands contain wheat starch.

Courtesy of Shelley Case, RD, author of *Gluten-Free Diet: A Comprehensive Resource Guide;* Medical Advisory Board Member–Celiac Disease Foundation; Gluten Intolerance Group; and Canadian Celiac Association

Table 6.4 Notes for Table 6.1 on Foods to Avoid

Food Category	Food Products	Notes
Milk and Dairy	Malted milk	Contains malt powder derived from malted barley.
Grains and Starches	Semolina	A coarsely ground grain (usually made from the refined portion of durum wheat) that can be used to make porridge or pasta.
	Atta	A fine whole-meal flour made from low-gluten, soft, texturized wheat; used in Indian flatbread. Also known as chapati flour.
	Bulgur (burghul)	Quick-cooking form of whole wheat. The wheat kernels are parboiled (partially cooked), dried, and then cracked. Used in soups, pilafs, stuffing, and salads such as tabbouleh.
	Einkorn, emmer, farro, kamut, spelt	Types of wheat. Many "wheat-free" foods are made from these varieties of wheat, especially kamut and spelt. Remember that "wheat-free" does not always mean "gluten-free."
	Triticale	A cereal grain that is a cross between wheat and rye.
	Orzo	A type of pasta that is the size and shape of rice. Used in soups and as a substitute for rice.
	Matzo	Unleavened bread made with wheat flour and water that comes in thin sheets. Used primarily during Passover.
	Matzo meal	Ground matzo.
	Matzo balls	Dumplings made of matzo meal, which is not gluten free. However, they can be made with potato flour, which is gluten free.
	Couscous	Granules of semolina (made from durum wheat) that are precooked and dried. Cooked couscous is served hot or cold as a main dish or salad ingredient.

	Tabbouleh	A salad usually made with bulgur wheat or couscous, which are not gluten free. Can also be made with quinoa, which is gluten free.
Meats and Alternatives	Fu	A dried gluten product derived from wheat and sold as thin sheets or thick, round cakes. Used as a protein supplement in Asian dishes such as soups and vegetables.
	Seitan	A meatlike food derived from wheat gluten used in many vegetarian dishes. Sometimes called "wheat meat."
Others	Licorice	Regular licorice contains wheat flour.
	Potato chips	Some brands of plain potato chips contain added wheat flour and/or wheat starch.
	Cereal- and malt-based beverages	Contain malted barley or other grains such as wheat or rye; examples are Postum and Ovaltine.
	Beer, ale, and lager	Basic ingredients include malted barley, hops (a type of flower), yeast, and water. As this mixture is only fermented and not distilled, it contains varying levels of gluten.
	Malt vinegar	Made from malted barley. As this vinegar is only fermented and not distilled, it contains varying levels of gluten.
	Soy sauce	Many brands are a combination of soy and wheat.
	Brewer's yeast	A dried, inactive yeast that is a bitter by-product of the brewing industry. It is not commonly used as a flavoring agent in foods. ELISA tests are unable to accurately confirm the amount of residual gluten in this type of yeast.

Courtesy of Shelley Case, RD, author of *Gluten-Free Diet: A Comprehensive Resource Guide*; Medical Advisory Board Member–Celiac Disease Foundation; Gluten Intolerance Group; and Canadian Celiac Association your reaction for twenty-four hours. Keep doing this—even if it takes a bit longer than a week—to arrive at your own personal list of "safe" foods.

Gluten Sensitivity Without Clear-Cut Evidence of Celiac Sprue

Many people have found that they are clearly sensitive to gluten-containing foods and yet have normal blood tests for celiac sprue and may also have a normal biopsy of the small bowel. Nevertheless, such patients often experience relief of dyspeptic-type symptoms while on a gluten-free diet. They may have just a sensitivity to gluten, or they may have "latent celiac," especially if they have a family history. If you fall into this category, use the information and treatment plan in this chapter as if you had celiac sprue.

▶What if Changing Your Diet Doesn't Work?

If you have been diagnosed with celiac sprue, you have changed your diet accordingly, and at the end of four weeks you are still having symptoms, you may have "unresponsive celiac disease." There are several possible explanations for this impasse:

■ **"Hidden" gluten.** There could still be gluten in your diet or medications of which you are not aware. The best solution is close consultation with a registered dietitian or nutritionist to ferret out and eliminate the sources.

■ **Intestinal damage.** Rarely, a person's intestine has been so damaged that it does not heal after several months on a gluten-free diet. Such individuals cannot absorb the nutrients from food. In these situations, people may need to receive nutrients directly into their bloodstreams intravenously.

■ **Pancreatic insufficiency.** This is a condition that can occur in association with celiac sprue. The pancreas normally produces juices that help the digestive process. A pancreas that is not stimulated to produce the required amount of juices can contribute to the persistence of diarrhea and failure to gain weight. Treatment may require a prescription of pancreatic enzyme supplements.

■ **Lactose intolerance.** With sprue there is damage to the lining of the small bowel, and therefore, not enough of the enzyme *lactase* is produced to help you digest *lactose*, which is the sugar in milk and other dairy products. People with sprue who are also milk intolerant may not be able to drink milk until the lining of the bowel returns to, or toward, normal while on a strict gluten-free diet. The way to test this out, in consultation with your nutritionist or doctor, is to repeat the elimination period of the Four-Week Plan, focusing only on dairy products this time.

■ **Collagenous sprue.** This is a condition in which the biopsy specimen from the small intestine shows increased scar tissue in the lining, which may require special treatment, such as corticosteroids or immunosuppressive drugs.

■ **Microscopic colitis.** People with sprue have an increased likelihood of incurring this inflammatory disorder of the colon, which can be diagnosed by a colonoscopic examination and biopsies. This requires additional treatment even while being on a gluten-free diet. Such treatments have included bismuth preparations and discontinuing all nonsteroidal anti-inflammatory drugs (NSAIDs), such as ibuprofen.

■ **Ulcerative jejunoileitis.** A precursor to intestinal lymphoma, ulcerative jejunoileitis is a condition in which people with celiac sprue develop ulcers in the small bowel that frequently do not respond to a gluten-free diet alone.

■ **T cell enteropathy, which can lead to lymphoma.** Celiac sprue puts people at increased risk of developing this premalignant or malignant condition, requiring further treatment with drugs that are used to treat gastrointestinal malignancies.

Hope Through Research

The celiac website of the National Institutes of Health (NIH) includes information that should give hope to anyone who is living with celiac sprue. The National Institute of Diabetes and Digestive and Kidney Disease, within the NIH (http://digestive.niddk.nih.gov/ddiseases/pubs/celiac), conducts and supports research on celiac disease. Current research is targeting the substances in gluten that are believed to be responsible for the destruction of the immune system function, as happens in celiac disease. In their search for treatments, researchers are engineering enzymes that they hope will block the effects of the proteins causing the damage.

Early diagnosis and treatment is, of course, the best way to help people with celiac sprue, so researchers are also developing programs and materials to raise awareness among health-care providers. As a patient, you can do your part by becoming better informed about celiac sprue and asking your doctor to provide you with information and direct you to resources, including support groups in your locale.

Points to Remember About Celiac Sprue

The same government source just cited also itemizes the salient points to remember, which comprise an at-a-glance profile as we sum up our discussion of celiac sprue:

- People with celiac sprue cannot tolerate gluten, a protein in wheat, rye, and barley (especially if they are exposed to wheat or other sources of gluten during the manufacturing process).
- Untreated celiac sprue damages the small intestine and interferes with nutrient absorption.
- Without treatment, people with celiac sprue can develop complications such as lymphoma, osteoporosis, anemia, and seizures.

- A person with celiac disease may or may not have symptoms.
- Diagnosis involves blood tests and a biopsy of the small intestine.
- Since celiac disease is hereditary, family members of a person with celiac disease may wish to be tested.
- Celiac disease is treated by eliminating all gluten from the diet; the gluten-free diet is a lifetime requirement.
- A dietitian can teach a person with celiac disease appropriate food selection, label reading, and other strategies to help manage the disease.

LIKE MOTHER, LIKE DAUGHTER

When Melinda S., thirty, came into my office, she was already confident of her diagnosis. "My pediatrician just told me my daughter has celiac sprue," she related. "I don't have any symptoms of it myself, so I know I don't have it, but I want you to do a blood test—just to be sure."

Let's review the lessons of this chapter before proceeding: When people with celiac sprue eat foods containing gluten, the breakdown products during digestion alter the lining of the small bowel and trigger an immune response that breeds further damage. This is considered an autoimmune disorder, in that the body is being stimulated to attack a part of itself—the lining of the small intestine. Gluten is a protein in wheat, rye, barley, and malt. It is also often used as a coating for vitamins and medicines, as well as a stabilizer in processed foods and bottled sauces.

Now, before ordering that blood test, I questioned Melinda about her medical and dietary history. This is what I found out: She had occasional diarrhea, but it was always associated with drinking beer—which contains a fair amount of gluten, owing to the malt ingredient. "Also, I always feel bloated when I eat bread and pizza," she admitted, "so, I just don't eat those foods much. I do like beer, however—I'm Irish, you know."

This was a highly relevant fact, since celiac sprue is much more common in people of northern European ancestry—in particular, Ireland. "Tell me about your parents," I prompted. It turns out that both her parents were born in Northern Ireland.

Celiac sprue also runs in families. If you have a first-order relative—mother, father, sister, brother, daughter, or son—you are five to ten times more likely to have the condition yourself.

Despite what Melinda believed about herself, not only did she have symptoms of celiac sprue, but also she had at least one close relative—her daughter—with the condition, as well as Irish ancestry. A test confirmed that Melinda had celiac sprue–related autoantibodies in her blood, and a later biopsy of her small intestine revealed damage consistent with celiac sprue. (Refer to Figure 6.1.)

In line with Melinda's approach, half of all people newly diagnosed with celiac sprue do not initially tell their doctors about the symptoms, especially gastrointestinal symptoms, they are having, probably because they do not consider them significant. Don't suffer in silence: if you experience abdominal bloating, cramps, and diarrhea, especially after consuming gluten-containing foods—or beer!—ask your doctor to test you for celiac sprue. Also be aware that about 2 to 4 percent of people who are initially diagnosed with irritable bowel syndrome turn out to have celiac sprue when the appropriate tests are done.

As soon as Melinda learned of her own diagnosis, dealing with celiac sprue transformed into a family project, since it was clear that gluten-containing foods were causing the symptoms in both mother and daughter. Instead of having to use the Four-Week Plan to test and eliminate foods, she and her daughter explored gluten-free foods, recipes, and websites. They bought cookbooks and a bread machine and began baking their own gluten-free bread, cakes, and muffins. At the same time, they did implement the methods of eating suggested in the Four-Week Plan, including calm, slow mealtimes and sufficient chewing for every bite. "Life is a little more complicated now," says Melinda, "but we both feel a lot better without those symptoms!"

Chapter 7

Diabetes

I f you are one of the millions of people living with diabetes, chances are that you are also having some problems with your digestion. About 80 percent of people with diabetes either have or will develop troublesome gastrointestinal symptoms. In this chapter, I will review some diabetes facts and tell you how diabetes can cause GI symptoms. I will also give you a Four-Week Plan for healthy digestion with diabetes.

Diabetes Facts

Diabetes is a disorder of the way our bodies use food for energy, so it is closely related to digestion. In your stomach and intestines, almost everything you eat is broken down into a sugar called glucose, which is the "fuel" our bodies use in order to function. When food is digested, the glucose passes into the blood. A hormone called insulin then moves the glucose out of the blood and into all the cells of the body, which use this fuel to do their jobs. Normally, when you eat, this process triggers an organ called the pancreas to produce just the right amount of insulin to transport the glucose out of the blood and into the cells.

If you have diabetes, however, either your pancreas produces little or no insulin (type 1 diabetes) or your cells do not respond properly to the insulin that is produced (type 2 diabetes). Without the glucose-transporting function of insulin, the glucose builds up in the blood and eventually overflows into the urine, passing out of the body. The body loses its main source of fuel, leading to a cluster of detrimental health effects, and the high level of glucose in the blood ("high blood sugar") causes additional problems. This book directly addresses only the *digestive* consequences of diabetes.

In the United States alone, an estimated 20.8 million people —7 percent of the population—have diabetes. Of these, some 6.2 million have not yet been diagnosed. Untreated diabetes can have serious health consequences, so if you have not been diagnosed with diabetes and are experiencing any of the symptoms listed in the accompanying sidebar, please see your doctor to request a diabetes test. If, on the other hand, you already know you have diabetes, the "Red Flags" sidebar farther along will alert you as to when it is incumbent to seek medical attention.

DIABETES SYMPTOMS

The following symptoms may indicate that you have diabetes. Then again, some people with diabetes have no symptoms at all. It is a good idea to discuss your risk factors with your doctor.

- Increased thirst and urination, especially increased urination at night*
- Constant hunger*
- Weight loss, in spite of good appetite and increased food intake
- Blurred vision
- Extreme fatigue
- Slow healing of wounds or sores
- New onset of numbness and tingling in the feet and legs
- New onset of unexplained diarrhea or constipation

*The three "P" warning signs of diabetes are polyphagia (increased appetite), polydipsia (increased thirst), and polyuria (increased urine output).

Diabetes and Digestion

If you know you have diabetes, it is of course important to work with your physician to keep your blood sugar levels under control. Even if you do this, however, you might still have problems such as diarrhea, constipation, difficulty swallowing, nausea, and feelings of bloating and discomfort. While most of these symptoms can be managed initially using the Four-Week Plan, you should seek immediate medical attention for any of the diabetes "red flag" symptoms listed in this section.

Diabetes can cause digestion problems in several different ways.

"Sugarless" Foods

As revealed in Chapter 2, sorbitol (a type of sugar alcohol, which is a potent laxative) is often present in the so-called sugarless foods recommended for people with diabetes. These include dietetic gum, candies, jams, pancake syrup, ice cream, gelatin desserts, and other foods. As opposed to being "sugarless," these foods actually contain sugar compounds that are not absorbed into your body! Read labels carefully, and be on the alert for sorbitol and other sugar alcohols.

Diabetes Nerve Damage

Levels of blood glucose that are too high can, over a period of years, damage the blood vessels that bring oxygen to the nerves, which in turn causes damage to the nerves they supply. Blood glucose that is too high can also injure the covering of the nerves themselves. Both of these kinds of damage may stop nerves from sending messages to the muscles and organs of the body, or they may cause the nerves to send the messages too slowly or at the wrong time.

Autonomic Neuropathy. What does nerve damage have to do with digestion? The autonomic nervous system controls activities in

DIABETES AND DIGESTION: RED FLAGS

If you have diabetes and experience any of the following symptoms, seek medical attention:

- Difficulty and/or pain in swallowing
- Persistent nausea or vomiting
- Persistent inability to eat a normal-size meal (early satiety), especially with weight loss
- Abdominal bloating and distension after a meal, which may indicate delayed stomach emptying
- Persistent diarrhea for a few months—even if it is intermittent
- Fecal incontinence (losing stool in the underwear); this can be an embarrassing symptom, but it is treatable, so do not hesitate to discuss it with your doctor (Do not describe it as "just diarrhea" and expect your doctor to give you a medicine to "stop the diarrhea.")
- Diabetic foods are often labeled dietetic, and the terms *diabetic* and *dietetic* are interchangeable.

your body without your even being aware of it. These activities include your heartbeat, your breathing, and your digestion, all of which go on even when you are asleep. When high blood glucose levels damage the autonomic nerves leading to the intestines and other parts of the digestive system, food passes through the system either too slowly (causing constipation) or too quickly (causing diarrhea). This is called *autonomic neuropathy*.

Slow Stomach Emptying. The condition in which nerve damage causes the stomach to empty too slowly is called slow stomach emptying or slow gastric emptying, or, more technically, *gastroparesis*. Damage to nerves in the stomach means that the stomach is not sending food promptly on its way to the intestines to be digested. If blood sugar levels exceed 200 milligrams per deciliter, the emptying of the stomach is also slowed. This slow movement of food can, as explained in Chapter 5, lead to bloating, nausea, discomfort, and gas. To compound the problem, gastroparesis also makes it harder to keep blood glucose levels under control.

Pancreatic Insufficiency

The pancreas is the organ that is most affected by diabetes, since it is the organ that produces insulin. The pancreas has another important digestion function as well: it produces the "digestive juices" that help break down the complex sugars, fats, and proteins in food into smaller products that can be more readily absorbed. Diabetes can alter the production of these digestive juices, resulting not only in abnormal absorption of the food breakdown products but also in the loss of calories, diarrhea, and, eventually, weight loss.

Bacterial Overgrowth in the Small Intestine

As explained in Chapter 2, abnormal growth and persistence of bacteria can interfere with digestive processes and thus cause decreased absorption of the nutrients in food. Both diarrhea and weight loss can result. Ordinarily, the upper small bowel is sterile (few bacteria are present). However, in people with diabetes, especially those who have nerve damage to the bowel, e.g., resultant autonomic neuropathy and slowed transit of food through the small intestine, bacteria can accumulate in the small bowel and interfere with the absorption of nutrients. Your doctor should be able to diagnose this condition with appropriate tests and treat it with carefully selected antibiotics.

Other Conditions

Even if you know you have diabetes, you may also have other conditions at the same time that can affect your digestion and bowel habits, such as celiac sprue (see Chapter 6) or irritable bowel syndrome (see Chapter 2). It is important for your doctor, knowing that you have diabetes, to check you for *all* the possible causes of your gastrointestinal symptoms.

▶Your Initial Four-Week Plan for Diabetes Digestion Problems

Digestion problems related to diabetes require a slight variation of our Four-Week Plan, involving your health-care team. You can begin your Food and Symptom Log in week one, but at the same time, you need to work with your physician to make sure that your blood sugar is under the best possible control. Having blood sugar levels consistently higher than 200 milligrams per deciliter can result in both decreased emptying of the stomach and difficult-to-control diabetes.

Accordingly, during weeks two and three, and especially if your GI symptoms persist, I encourage consultation with a gastroenterology specialist, who might well take an additional medical history from you to determine exactly what is causing your symptoms. If, for example, you were having symptoms of gastroparesis (slow stomach emptying), I would order special tests that measure the rate of emptying. Normally, half of your meal should leave your stomach within one hour.

The actions you take during week three—such as eliminating foods—should likewise be done in consultation with your doctor, always keeping a close eye on your blood sugar levels. If your problem is slow stomach emptying, for example, you could use this week to eliminate fatty, heavy foods, such as steak, which slow the stomach down. You should also be eating smaller, more frequent meals. In addition, ask your doctor about medicines—called prokinetics—that speed up the stomach; these are taken thirty to forty-five minutes before a major meal. Normalizing the rate of stomach emptying will make it easier to control your diabetes.

If your problems are related to diarrhea or constipation, work with your physician to adjust your diet in line with the suggestions in earlier chapters. No matter what you do, place a premium on keeping your blood sugar under good control. For people with diabetes, this means that the HgbA1c (hemoglobin A1c) is maintained at a value of between 6 and 7.

Take a Bottom-Up Approach

During week four and beyond, as you consolidate your dietary changes, the advice for people with diabetes is consistent with what Harvard nutrition experts recommend for everyone else:

- Achieve and maintain a healthy weight.
- Include plenty of fruits and vegetables in your diet (but limit white potatoes).
- Reduce unhealthy fats in your diet, and replace them with healthy fats.
- Choose healthy complex carbohydrates over refined sugars and refined starches.
- Increase the amount of fiber you eat.
- Opt for healthier proteins, such as beans, nuts, fish, and poultry, instead of red meat.
- If you drink alcohol, do so in moderation.
- Limit your salt intake.
- Get enough calcium (1,000 milligrams per day).
- Take a multivitamin each day.

The relationship of these elements is summed up in the Healthy Eating Pyramid, developed by Walter C. Willett, chair of the department of nutrition at the Harvard School of Public Health and a professor of medicine at Harvard Medical School. (See Figure 7.1.) This pyramid, which differs significantly from the USDA Food Pyramid, is based on findings from well-developed scientific studies.

Obviously, if you have celiac sprue, you must avoid all gluten-containing grains. There are, however, several other nutritious grains that do not contain gluten, and the websites suggested in Chapter 6 can give you more information about where to find them.

In the past, people with diabetes were advised to avoid all sugar, but that restriction has been loosened. According to the American Diabetes Association: "Now experts agree that you can eat foods with sugar as long as you work them into your meal plan as you

Figure 7.1 **Healthy Eating Pyramid**

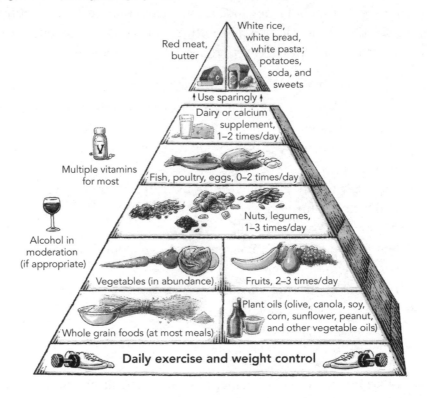

As you embark on your Four-Week Plan for diabetes digestion problems, this handy guide will help. Focus *most* on daily exercise and weight control, choosing more whole-grain foods, plant and vegetable oils, fruits, vegetables, nuts, legumes, lean poultry, and fish. *Eat only sparingly*: red meat, white rice, white bread, potatoes, pasta, and sweets.

Source: Adapted from *Eat, Drink, and Be Healthy* by Walter C. Willett with Patrick J. Skerrett, Free Press, 2005.

would any other carb-containing food. The same guidelines apply to other sweeteners with calories, including brown sugar, honey, and molasses."

Vigilance Brings Rewards

I caution you again: read labels carefully, and beware of so-called diabetic sugar and fat substitutes, such as Splenda, and sugar alcohols such as sorbitol, isomalt, maltitol, mannitol, and xylitol. These substances—which do not actually contain alcohol—are poorly absorbed sugars that can cause diarrhea. They are called sugar alcohols because of their chemical structure.

Diabetes is a complicating factor as you strive for healthy digestion. Not only is what you eat important, but also you must be conscious of the danger of gaining too much weight—which is a major risk factor for type 2 diabetes—as well as the necessity of adding exercise to your daily routine. All of these behaviors will help not only your diabetes but also every other part of your health. If you work closely with your physician, your GI specialist, and perhaps a nutritionist, you might be able to control your blood sugar levels without medication, have more energy, and still be able to enjoy your food!

THE "SUGARLESS" PARADOX

Gerard R., sixty, had always exhibited excellent health. He played golf on weekends, enjoyed fine dining, and had never experienced any trouble with his digestion. Until now. He came to see me because of debilitating diarrhea. He remarked, "Having to use the bathroom so often is interrupting my workday, my social life, and, most important, my golf game!"

The most significant recent change in Gerard's life had been a diagnosis of type 2 diabetes six months previously. "I was shocked," he confided as I took his medical history during our initial visit. "My doctor told me I had to radically change my diet—no more of my favorite desserts and snacks." Giving up cookies, candies, and especially chocolate was hard for him, he said. He added, "I also had to start a real exercise program, not just weekend golf."

In order to rule out common causes of diarrhea, I arranged for a colon examination (he had never had one), as well as tests for celiac sprue (gluten intolerance). All tests came back negative. So, at our next visit, I asked him about any changes in his diet. At first, he shook his head. "Except for cutting out all my favorite treats, there has been no change," he said, somewhat sadly. I asked, "How have you managed to cut out all those sweets?" He replied that he had (rather cleverly, he thought) substituted sugarless gum, mints, and candies. "Whenever I feel the urge to buy a candy bar, I pop some sugarless gum into my mouth," he told me proudly. "I haven't had a candy bar in months." When I pressed him about how much of the gum he had been chewing, he said he went through about one pack a day.

Here was the clue to his diarrhea. I enlightened Gerard to the cruel fact that sugarless gum, mints, and other so-called diabetic foods such as "sugarless" jams, pancake syrups, and sugar-free packaged desserts are not sugarless at all, in that they contain significant amounts of sorbitol, which is a sugar alcohol. Everyone, not just people with diabetes, should beware of sugar substitutes in addition to sorbitol, such as isomalt, maltitol, mannitol, and xylitol. These do not actually contain alcohol, but are poorly absorbed sugars. All of these substitutes can be potent causes of diarrhea in many hapless people.

Gerard and I pored over the labels of some of the "sugarless" foods he had been eating, and he was taken aback by the amount of sugar alcohols listed. "I guess I have to be more vigilant about what I am putting in my mouth," he commented. "The consequences of being careless just aren't worth it!"

Gerard called me just one week later to report that he had ostracized all sugar and fat substitute products from his diet. "I'm munching on raw vegetables instead," he told me, "and it's not too bad, especially since I am completely back to my normal bowel habits. I'm looking forward to a nice, long round of golf this weekend!"

Chapter 8

For Women Only

If you are a woman, you are more prone than a man to have at least one of the digestive problems already discussed in this book: irritable bowel syndrome (see Chapter 2). You are also much more susceptible to the digestive and other effects of alcohol than are men. Please see the sidebar that follows for the recommended alcohol intake limits for women. (Fuller treatment appears in Chapter 5.)

Your female hormones also predispose you to other potential digestion problems. You are most likely all too familiar with the changes that occur in your body each month just before and during your menstrual flow, making you feel tired, bloated, and irritable. What you may not realize is that these changes—as well as those that occur during pregnancy and menopause—are the result of the complex and constantly changing balance of your female hormones: estrogen and progesterone. Changes in these hormones can also affect your digestion. So, if you have digestion problems for which you have not yet found explanations, this chapter is meant for you, and if you have a teenage daughter, the information may be useful for her as well. Figure 8.1 is provided as a reference.

Figure 8.1 **Digestive Organs That Respond to Hormonal Changes**

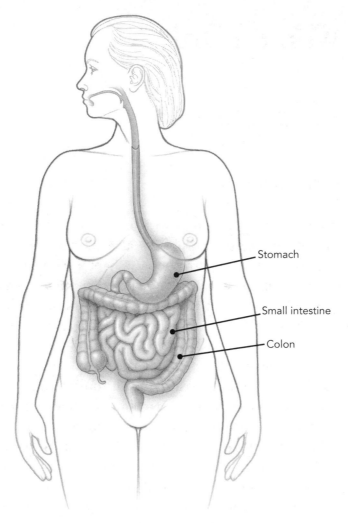

Stomach

Small intestine

Colon

Monthly hormonal changes, as well as pregnancy and menopause, can affect the digestive organs.

▶Your Monthly Period and Digestion

Each month, your body prepares for a possible pregnancy. An egg is released from one of your ovaries, and the lining of your uterus begins to thicken, just in case the egg is fertilized and you become

> ## RECOMMENDED ALCOHOL INTAKE FOR WOMEN WHO ARE NOT PREGNANT
>
> If you regularly exceed the recommended limits of one unit per day or seven units per week, I encourage you to discuss your alcohol intake with your doctor.
>
> One unit of alcohol is equal to ten grams, which is the amount in each of the following servings:
>
> - One ounce of whiskey
> - One twelve-ounce bottle of beer
> - One four-ounce glass of wine

pregnant. This process is orchestrated by a complex balancing of estrogen and progesterone. If the egg is not fertilized and you do not become pregnant, your body then undergoes a different process of hormonal changes that cause the egg, as well as the newly built-up lining of your uterus, to pass out of your body during a menstrual period.

In addition to fertility, the monthly fluctuations in the levels of estrogen and progesterone can have digestive consequences, including diarrhea, constipation, upset stomach, bloating, and food cravings. The following sections capsulize some common digestion problems linked to hormonal changes in women.

GERD (Gastroesophageal Reflux Disease) and Heartburn

One of the most significant digestive consequences of the menstrual cycle is an increase in the transient (short-lived) inappropriate relaxation of the gastroesophageal sphincter. This can result from the increased levels of progesterone that occur just before you have your period. Recalling the presentation in Chapter 4, a circular band of muscle called the gastroesophageal sphincter controls the "doorway" between your stomach and your esophagus (the tube connecting your mouth and your stomach). When this muscle relaxes inappropriately—such as well after a meal, when it normally remains closed—the contents of the stomach can move back up into the esophagus, causing discomfort and the sensation known as heartburn.

If this happens only occasionally before your period, you can follow the food suggestions in Chapter 4. You may also occasionally seek relief from over-the-counter heartburn remedies, but this should be done only in consultation with your doctor and for no longer than a few days. If symptoms persist beyond your period, use the GERD Four-Week Plan.

Irritable Bowel Syndrome

In addition to heartburn or GERD, monthly hormonal changes can make symptoms of irritable bowel syndrome (IBS) worse. These symptoms may include painful diarrhea, bloating, mucus in the stool, stomach cramps, and gas. Please see Chapter 2 for details about the diagnosis and treatment of IBS, as well as the IBS Four-Week Plan. It is also a good idea to discuss with your physician the possible connection between IBS symptoms and your menstrual period.

Endometriosis

While endometriosis is a disease of the uterus, it can also have an effect on your digestion. Endometriosis occurs when tissue that belongs inside the uterus "escapes" out into the abdomen and grows there, causing scarring and pain in the abdominal organs and interfering with digestion. Digestive symptoms caused by endometriosis include pain in the abdomen, as well as discomfort during bowel movements or urination. This condition must be diagnosed, evaluated, and treated by a gynecologist. Endometriosis can cause significant gastrointestinal (GI) symptoms such as cramping, lower-abdominal pain, and alteration of bowel habits (constipation or diarrhea) and may mimic other GI disorders such as IBS. As such, it should always be considered in any evaluation of digestive symptoms that are worsened during the menstrual cycle.

MONTHLY MISERIES

The patient, Diana G., a woman in her mid-thirties, was not quite sure why she was in my office. "My husband wanted me to see you," she said. "I have a family history of colon cancer, hypertension, and diabetes, and he wanted me to have a complete exam." A physical examination was entirely normal. I asked her if she herself was concerned about any health problems. At first, she said no; this was all her husband's idea. But, well, there was this one thing . . . she does get a bit irritable around the time of her monthly period. "Tell me more about this," I encouraged her.

"It probably gets a bit hard for my husband every month," she admitted. "The week before and during my period, I'm always uncomfortable." She added quickly, "But the reason I'm here has nothing to do with my period." "Actually," I said, "the hormonal changes that happen at this time every month affect the smooth muscles of the digestive tract. Such changes can slow the stomach down, aggravating dyspepsia, reflux, and heartburn, as well as diarrhea. Some women even have bloating and distension and loose bowel movements at the same time."

She stared at me and asked, "How could you possibly know what I've been going through, when I didn't tell you?" I assured her that there was nothing mysterious. These are common problems affecting many of my women patients who have not yet reached menopause. (Menopause itself, especially if the woman has had a hysterectomy, can trigger constipation or make it worse.)

"Is there anything I can do to ease these symptoms?" she asked. Together, we went through the Four-Week Plans for dyspepsia, diarrhea, and GERD. Over the next few months, she identified the kind of diet that worked best for her just before and during her periods. It featured bland foods, vegetables, and rice, along with eating smaller meals. For short-term alleviation of dyspepsia symptoms, she will sometimes use over-the-counter medicines.

Several months later, I heard from her. "I now have what I call my 'special monthly foods,'" she announced. "Both my husband and I are much happier these days!"

▶Pregnancy and GI Problems

If you are pregnant, you certainly have many more things than digestion to think about! Nevertheless, being pregnant does make you more susceptible to certain gastrointestinal problems, and that is what I hope to enlighten you about here. For some of these problems, you can use the specific Four-Week Plans described in previous chapters, since these plans generally involve only dietary and lifestyle changes and do not require medication that may be harmful to your baby. For other conditions, you will need to consult with your obstetrician about treatments that are safe for both you and your baby.

During pregnancy, treatment of gastrointestinal problems is complicated, because one wants to be sure that the baby is protected as much as possible from the side effects of medication or the potential dangers of surgical procedures. Therefore, the goal of your obstetrician will be to control your symptoms as safely as feasible, while minimizing the need for medication or surgery until after your baby is born. Of course, some emergency situations, such as appendicitis, will require surgery, but those kinds of events are outside the scope of this book.

GI RED FLAGS FOR PREGNANT WOMEN

The following digestive symptoms require immediate medical attention during pregnancy:

- Vomiting that is so severe that it leads to dehydration and weight loss
- Diarrhea or constipation accompanied by fever, abdominal pain, tenderness, or a distended abdomen unrelated to the pregnancy
- Blood in the stool
- Severe abdominal pain accompanied by fever

Nausea and Vomiting During Pregnancy

As unpleasant as "morning sickness" may be, there is some evidence that nausea during the first trimester is actually a good sign. Nausea and vomiting during pregnancy have been associated with *lower* risks of miscarriage, of low infant birth weight, and of preterm birth, possibly because these symptoms indicate

TREATMENT OF NAUSEA AND VOMITING DURING PREGNANCY

If you are vomiting so severely that you are becoming dehydrated and are losing weight, seek immediate medical attention. Otherwise, the following suggestions may aid in relieving nausea during pregnancy, but always check first with your physician and obstetrician.

■ Avoid fatty foods, which can delay stomach emptying.

■ Eat small, frequent meals of bland carbohydrates (starches such as noodles, potatoes, and rice), chicken, and fish.

■ If your vomiting is severe, try taking small sips of salty liquids such as sports beverages or broth. Avoid juices, as well as creamy or dairy beverages, because they make symptoms worse.

■ Acupressure, often performed with the use of wristbands (Sea-bands is a well-known brand) worn continuously for a period of a few days, followed by a hiatus of few days, may help. This treatment is noninvasive, and many women report a reduction in the number of episodes of nausea. (This response may be partly due to the placebo effect—but whatever works, works!)

■ Recent research also supports the use of pyridoxine (vitamin B_6) for control of nausea symptoms, and another small trial comparing 1.05 grams of ginger daily for three weeks versus 75 milligrams of pyridoxine found a similar modest benefit in reducing symptoms of nausea.

that the proper hormonal and physical changes needed in your body for a successful pregnancy have been achieved. Almost 80 percent of women experience nausea during the first trimester, and for some, this is the symptom that leads to the diagnosis of pregnancy.

In a study of 160 pregnant women, led by Jaya Agrawal and Sonia Friedman (in the forthcoming book *Current Gastroenterology, Hepatology, and Endoscopy*; McGraw-Hill), 80 percent of the subjects said that the nausea lasted all day, so the usage "morning sickness" can be misleading. The average duration of the nausea was thirty-five days, and only half of the women had relief of nausea by the fourteenth week of pregnancy, though symptoms disappeared in 90 percent of women by week twenty-two.

GERD and Heartburn During Pregnancy

Heartburn symptoms, attributed to gastroesophageal reflux, occur in nearly two-thirds of pregnancies, with symptoms becoming more common and more severe during the third trimester, possibly because of increased abdominal pressure as the baby grows. If you did not have GERD before you became pregnant, there is a good chance that your symptoms will disappear after delivery, although some women report that their symptoms persist. If you had a history of GERD before your pregnancy, you are at higher risk to have it during pregnancy. Other risk factors include multiple births and your age—if you are below age forty, you may be more likely to have GERD during pregnancy.

Constipation During Pregnancy

During pregnancy, it is common to experience constipation or, for some women, a worsening of chronic constipation. For one thing, you may be drinking less fluid, perhaps because of nausea and vomiting, and may not be sufficiently hydrated. Likewise, many pregnant women are prescribed iron supplements, which can also contribute to constipation. Finally, if you are exercising less and

TREATMENT OF GERD AND HEARTBURN
DURING PREGNANCY

To avoid risks to the baby, lifestyle modifications should be your first choice of treatment for GERD and heartburn during pregnancy. Referring back to Chapter 4, this means avoiding alcohol, caffeine, mint, chocolate, tobacco, and fatty and spicy foods. Also, do not eat late-night meals—that is, within three hours before you go to bed. Another way to prevent nighttime symptoms is to raise the head of your bed by putting blocks under the legs. Simply using more pillows will not help, since that raises only your head, and you need to also raise your chest.

If none of these measures works, you can discuss medications, such as calcium-based antacids and proton pump inhibitors, with your physician. Do not take any medications on your own, and be especially wary of antacids containing magnesium when you are pregnant.

spending more time resting, your digestion may be slowed, and this can lead to constipation. In addition to these lifestyle factors, hormonal changes such as increased progesterone and estrogen are thought to retard the digestion process.

Diarrhea During Pregnancy

I stated previously that symptoms of irritable bowel syndrome may be exacerbated during pregnancy, but even if you do not have IBS, you may have diarrhea, although the causes may be the same as for nonpregnant women. These causes include viral infections such as rotavirus and Norwalk virus, which are associated with large-volume, watery diarrhea that eventually will end on its own as your body fights the infection. Diarrhea caused by bacteria (as opposed to a virus) often produces more frequent stools of small volume, abdominal pain, occasional fever, and blood and white blood cells, i.e., leukocytes in the stool.

TREATMENT OF CONSTIPATION DURING PREGNANCY

Seek immediate medical attention if you have constipation during pregnancy that is accompanied by fever, abdominal pain, tenderness, or a distended belly unrelated to the pregnancy. Otherwise, the treatment of constipation in pregnancy is similar to its treatment in nonpregnant women, so you can use the Four-Week Plan for constipation described in Chapter 3.

Your first line of treatment should be eating more fiber, which is the safest way to alleviate constipation. Here is a reminder of suggested high-fiber foods:

- Fruits—especially peaches, pears, cherries, apples, orange juice, and apple juice
- Brassica vegetables—such as broccoli, asparagus, cauliflower, brussels sprouts, and cabbage
- Beans
- Whole-grain breads
- Coffee
- Tea
- Salads—especially celery, which is high in fiber

If eating more fiber does not help, you should discuss other safe options with your obstetrician, including psyllium, calcium polycarbophil, and methylcellulose, which are bulk laxatives and can be used as an alternative or in addition to fiber-rich foods. These products should be diluted and taken with food during meals. The laxative effect of these supplements may be delayed for days, and you should also be aware that fiber can cause bloating and gas that may persist for two to four weeks. It is important to drink at least one and a half quarts of fluid a day (at least six glasses) when you add fiber to your diet.

Your doctor may also wish to perform tests to determine how much time it takes for food to progress through your system. These tests are described in Chapter 3.

) **TREATMENT OF DIARRHEA DURING PREGNANCY**

There is usually no need to discuss diarrhea with your doctor if it is occasional, is clearly food related, and stops on its own. *However, do seek immediate medical attention if your diarrhea is severe, leads to dehydration or weight loss, is bloody, or is associated with high fevers, or if it persists for more than forty-eight hours without improvement.*

Otherwise, please consult Chapter 2 for dietary suggestions, along with the Four-Week Plan for diarrhea. As a reminder, avoid sugary foods, as well as so-called sugarless gum, candies, mints, syrups, and desserts; they usually contain high amounts of sorbitol and other sugar alcohols, which are potent laxatives. Check labels carefully! Also avoid high-fiber foods (listed in the "Treatment of Constipation" sidebar), and soothe your stomach with low-fiber foods such as white rice, white bread, bananas, potatoes, and well-cooked fish, chicken, broiled meats, and veal.

Be sure to return to a balanced diet of fruits, vegetables, and whole grains, as well as meats and fish, as soon as possible. Your baby and you will both benefit!

Irritable Bowel Syndrome During Pregnancy

IBS—which can include diarrhea and constipation, as well as other symptoms—is common in pregnancy, partly because it is a common syndrome in women of childbearing age and partly because pregnancy seems to make associated gastrointestinal symptoms worse. Many women experience either an increase in constipation or, conversely, an increase in stool frequency. By the same token, while abdominal pain, bloating, flatulence, and nausea can also worsen during pregnancy, partly as the result of female hormones acting on the digestive tract, for some women, IBS symptoms may actually improve.

If you had IBS before you were pregnant and are experiencing the same or worse symptoms now, be sure to let your doctor know.

TREATMENT OF IBS DURING PREGNANCY

By far the safest way to treat IBS during pregnancy is through what you eat. Please see Chapter 2 for dietary suggestions if you have diarrhea, and Chapter 3 if you have constipation. Chapter 2 also contains details about IBS symptoms and diagnosis. In addition, your doctor may prescribe fiber supplements, which are used to treat both diarrhea and constipation associated with IBS. Although these may lead to bloating and gas that may persist for four to six weeks, the effects will decrease over time.

Symptoms that suggest IBS during pregnancy include some combination of pain, gas, irregular bowel movements, and mucus in stools, especially if your symptoms are more pronounced after you eat and are relieved after you move your bowels.

Gallstones (Biliary Disease) During Pregnancy

Hormonal changes and other factors such as weight gain may predispose you to develop gallstones during pregnancy. These small "stones" come from bile that is stored in the gallbladder and that has been altered during the pregnancy so that it is more likely to coalesce. Gallstone formation also can be the result of too much cholesterol in the bile, or of a deficiency of bile salts, which act to keep the cholesterol from forming stones. Another known contributor is slow emptying of the gallbladder, which is a frequent occurrence in pregnancies.

Gallstones can be located either in the gallbladder itself or, infrequently, in the bile ducts that are connected to it. Gallstone pain is typically felt in the right upper part of the abdomen, just below the rib cage. It may come in waves of pain of increasing and decreasing severity. The pain may last from thirty minutes to a few hours, is likely to occur after meals, and may even awaken you from sleep. The rather sharp pain then may blend into a dull ache, and you may also feel discomfort in your back or in your shoulder.

Gallstone pain may be triggered by fatty foods and large meals. If you have any of the foregoing symptoms, especially after a heavy, fatty meal, and particularly if you have a fever, you should seek immediate medical attention.

OVERCOMING AN EMBARRASSING PROBLEM

The young mother, Samantha D., who was in my office was obviously having a hard time looking me in the eye. "I have had this nagging, persistent diarrhea ever since I gave birth to my third child four months ago," she said.

I suspected that the problem was worse than she was saying, so I tried to probe gently. "What was the delivery like?" I asked.

She looked fully at me for the first time. "The labor was very hard," she said. "The doctor had to use a forceps to get the baby out. Thank goodness he was OK! Which is more than I can say for me."

"Women who have forceps deliveries often have a problem with diarrhea afterward," I told her, "especially if this is not their first delivery. This is because the forceps can damage the anal sphincter, which is the muscle that holds stool inside your body until you are ready to let it out. In fact, some kind of damage to the anal sphincter happens in up to 70 percent of women who undergo forceps deliveries."

Samantha was looking at me intently now. "What does that mean?" she asked.

"For one thing, it means that women often lose their stool in their underwear before they make it to the bathroom," I answered. "This is really a very common problem, but most women are too embarrassed to discuss it with their doctors. This is too bad, since there is absolutely nothing to be embarrassed about. We know just what causes it, and we also know how to make it better."

She exhaled deeply, finally relaxing her body. "This is what is happening to me," she whispered. "I don't know what to do about it, especially having to take care of my children and a new baby." I explained to her the program of biofeedback and muscle training that we use to help people with this problem, and she eagerly asked when she could start.

Biofeedback gives you awareness of bodily functions that usually occur automatically, such as heart rate or muscle contractions. This training is a painless—and often enlightening—experience, during which the doctor will attach sensors to your skin and use a computer screen to show you changes in your muscle, brain wave, or heart activity. Biofeedback has been shown to be effective in retraining and strengthening the pelvic floor muscles to help control the anal sphincter and prevent the loss of stool.

Two months after starting the biofeedback program, Samantha called me. "It happens much less frequently now," she said happily, "especially if I follow your diarrhea food guidelines and watch what I eat. Now I can take my kids to the park without worrying!"

Menopause and Digestion

If you are either facing menopause (perimenopausal), in the middle of it, or postmenopausal, you may be having some related digestive problems. If you have undergone a hysterectomy, for example, you may have noticed increased problems with constipation. Statistics show that about 5 percent of women who have had hysterectomies experience constipation that is difficult to manage. If you notice the onset or worsening of constipation symptoms after a hysterectomy, be sure to inform your doctor, and be sure to drink enough fluids, eat the high-fiber foods listed in Chapter 3, and get regular exercise. Even just a daily walk can make a difference!

The news isn't all bad, by any means. Many women report that diarrhea and IBS symptoms tend to diminish after menopause, although this may not be the case for GERD and heartburn symptoms. A good general guideline for women at this stage—or any stage—of life is to maintain a healthy weight and a balanced diet, avoiding fatty foods and foods high in sugar. Equally important for digestive health, as well as overall body health, is sufficient exercise.

We thus come back to our first general premise: you cannot separate gastrointestinal health from overall health. Each of us must take some responsibility for our overall health and well-being.

Chapter 9

Communicating with Your Doctor

O ne of the underlying points I hope you have gleaned from this book is the significance of your own role in achieving healthy digestion. The Four-Week Plan will not work without you! While some gastrointestinal symptoms derive from genetic causes, disease, or structural problems, many are also linked to your lifestyle. Factors such as what you choose to eat or drink, the way in which you eat, and how much you eat are completely under your control, and they make a significant difference in your digestive health.

Of course, you are not in this alone. Your doctor is an important partner—but that is the key word: *partner*. This means that you and your doctor *both* play a role in determining whether and how your symptoms will improve. So, in this last chapter, I would like to share with you, from my perspective as a physician who has cared for thousands of patients, some suggestions of how best to communicate with your doctor regarding your digestive health.

History Lessons

The most important action you can take during your appointment with your doctor is to share information. Physicians, especially primary care doctors, often have limited time, so they will appreciate all of the specific information you can pass along about your symptoms and your lifestyle. This is where your Food and Symptom Log will be front and center. As you fill it in as part of your Four-Week Plan (as described in Chapter 1), not only will you be collecting valuable information to share with your doctor, but also you may begin to see a pattern yourself: When do your symptoms occur? What makes them worse? What makes them better?

When maintained in accordance with the guidelines in this book, your log will prove invaluable as a written record of all vitamins, medications, herbs, supplements, and over-the-counter products you have used, as well as their effects. It will also memorialize any candy, gum, or mints, as well as all beverages, that you've consumed, since even so-called sugarless foods have their risks, because of the laxative effect of sugar alcohols that they contain, such as sorbitol.

Part of sharing information is a detailed dietary history that goes beyond your Food and Symptom Log. When I teach medical students and residents, I always stress the importance of taking the time to elicit a detailed digestive and dietary history—including digestive problems in siblings, parents, and grandparents; long-term eating habits; medications; surgeries; previous digestive problems; and previous attempts to solve those problems.

If you notice that your doctor is not taking such a history, you might gently suggest that you share this information. Another approach is to write it down ahead of time and give it to your doctor. You could even mention this book and its emphasis on a detailed digestive and dietary history as part of any treatment plan.

This brings me to something *not* to do. While the Internet can be a valuable source of medical information, provided that the information comes from reputable sites (such as those specified in earlier chapters), it is not a bright idea to diagnose yourself. Diagnosis is the job of your doctor; this is what he or she is trained to do. If you come to your appointment armed with piles of articles and proclaiming what you think is wrong, you might risk putting a strain on your relationship with your doctor. Instead, I would advise asking open-ended questions, such as, "Do you think my diarrhea might be due to IBS?" Then listen carefully to the answers.

This does not mean that you should refrain from discussion! In fact, most doctors enjoy a lively give-and-take with their patients, and if you have certain treatment preferences, such as alternative therapies, you should feel free to say so. It is also important for your doctor to understand *your* personal perspective on your problem, how it is affecting your life and what it is preventing you from doing. You are a unique person, and no one is experiencing your digestive problems exactly as you are, so help your doctor get to know you better and understand your life.

▶Who Knew?

The details that you provide—as well as how you interpret the advice you receive— can have a profound effect on your treatment. Here are just two examples:

A woman came to the doctor because of problems with kidney stones, and her doctor advised her to increase her intake of fluids to a couple of liters of water a day. Several weeks later, she was back. The kidney stones had disappeared, but now she was having about ten loose bowel movements a day. The doctor was puzzled until she probed further: exactly *how* had her patient increased her fluid intake? It turned out that the woman had taken the advice a bit too enthusiastically. Instead of one to two liters of water a day, she had been drinking six to eight liters, and not just of water—she had added "vitamin water," sodas, and sport drinks, all of which contain large amounts of sugar. One sixteen-ounce soda, for example, contains forty grams of fructose, not to mention 160 calories. In 15 percent of healthy people, fructose and other sugars are poorly absorbed, resulting in diarrhea.

Another woman was having the opposite problem: constipation. It took several visits to successive doctors before her primary care doctor realized that she was on several medications—all prescribed by different doctors—that combined to slow the stomach down significantly, resulting in severe constipation. What were these medications? Antihistamines for nasal congestion, prescribed by her allergist; a calcium channel blocker to control hypertension, prescribed by her cardiologist; calcium for her bones, prescribed by her internist; and tricyclic antidepressants, prescribed by her psychiatrist. No one had told her of the potential digestive impact of each of these medications, not to mention the combined effects of all of them!

As the experiences of both of these patients suggest, *you* are a vital source of information to your doctor. Think of yourself as a medical detective: begin to notice *everything* that goes into your mouth. Then *write it down*, along with the effects on your digestion, and *share* this information with your doctor. Together with your doctor, you will find your personal pathway to healthy digestion.

· · · · · · · · · · · · · · · · · · ·

PART 2

Healthy Digestion Recipes

The following recipes are arranged under seven headings according to the conditions for which they are most beneficial. The sections feature recipes to improve the symptoms of diarrhea, constipation, GERD, dyspepsia, and celiac sprue; recipes that are useful for various combinations of those five and grouped in a category called "Recipes to Improve Multiple Conditions"; and, finally, recipes for diabetes.

Throughout all of the recipes, you will notice that certain ingredients have special symbols next to them. These symbols alert you that if you have the corresponding condition, such as celiac sprue or lactose intolerance, you should either eliminate this ingredient or use it with caution.

Happy cooking and eating!

KEY TO SYMBOLS IN RECIPES

* Avoid with celiac sprue disease, unless label clearly states "Certified gluten-free."
~ Avoid with dyspepsia.
+ Use with caution with dyspepsia.
■ Avoid with lactose intolerance.

▶Recipes to Improve Diarrhea Symptoms

Balsamic Marinated Pork Loin

1 1-pound boneless pork loin
½ cup balsamic vinegar
2 shallots, chopped ~
2 teaspoons minced garlic (about 4 cloves) ~
2 teaspoons dry mustard

Remove any visible fat from pork. Combine vinegar, shallots, garlic, and mustard in a bowl. Place pork in the bowl, cover, and refrigerate for 1 to 2 hours, turning pork occasionally to marinate all sides.

Preheat oven to 375°F. Remove pork from marinade (reserve), and place in a skillet over medium heat. Brown on all sides. Transfer pork to a casserole pan, and bake for about 15 to 20 minutes, until juices run clear and meat is white in center. While pork is cooking, pour reserved marinade into a saucepan, and simmer over medium-low heat until reduced by half. Serve marinade as sauce to accompany pork.

Makes 4 servings (¼ pound, uncooked, per serving)

Nutrition information per serving: Calories: 285; Total fat: 13.2 g;
    Saturated fat: 4.6 g; Trans fat: 0 g; Cholesterol: 69.7 mg; Sodium: 58 mg;
    Total carbohydrates: 15.5 g; Fiber: 0.2 g; Sugars: 6.4 g; Protein: 25.6 g

Beef Stew with Mushrooms and Onions

1 pound extra-lean (top or bottom round) stew beef

2 tablespoons whole-wheat flour *

2 teaspoons ground cumin *

1 teaspoon ground black pepper

1 tablespoon olive or canola oil

8 ounces white mushrooms, washed and sliced

8 ounces red or white pearl onions, peeled ~

1 teaspoon dried rosemary, * or 2 teaspoons fresh chopped

1 teaspoon minced garlic ~

½ cup red wine +

1 tablespoon red wine vinegar

1 cup low-sodium beef broth *

Remove any visible fat from beef cubes. Combine flour, cumin, and pepper in a bowl. Toss beef in flour mixture until well coated. Heat oil in a large skillet over medium heat. Add beef, and cook until brown on all sides. Add mushrooms, onions, rosemary, and garlic, and stir to combine. Reduce heat to low, and cook for 3 minutes. Add wine, and simmer until liquid is reduced by half. Stir in vinegar and broth. Cover and cook over very low heat for 2½ to 3 hours, until meat is tender.

Makes 4 servings

Nutrition information per serving: Calories: 211; Total fat: 8 g; Saturated fat: 2.1 g; Trans fat: 0 g; Cholesterol: 50 mg; Sodium: 81 mg; Total carbohydrates: 11.7 g; Fiber: 2 g; Sugars: 1.6 g; Protein: 27.7 g

Brown Basmati Rice Pilaf

1 tablespoon olive oil
½ cup diced red onion ~
3 cloves garlic, minced ~
2 bay leaves
2½ cups low-sodium chicken or vegetable broth *
1 cup brown basmati rice
4 green onions, sliced ~

Heat oil in a large skillet over low heat. Add onion and garlic, and
sauté until onion is translucent. Add bay leaves and broth, and
bring to a boil. Stir in rice, lower heat, and simmer for about 45
minutes, until cooked. Remove bay leaves. Stir green onions into
cooked rice mixture.

Makes 4 servings

Nutrition information per serving: Calories: 217; Total fat: 6.2 g; Saturated
fat: 0.7 g; Trans fat: 0 g; Cholesterol: 0 mg; Sodium: 48 mg; Total
carbohydrates: 36.5 g; Fiber: 2.7 g; Sugars: 2.2 g; Protein: 6.5 g

Spaghetti Salad

4 ounces whole-wheat spaghetti, broken into small pieces *

4 ounces low-fat mozzarella cheese, shredded + ▦

3 plum tomatoes, quartered and sliced +

4 green onions, sliced ~

1 cup artichoke hearts (frozen and thawed or canned in water), cut
   into small pieces

¼ cup diced red onion ~

¼ cup olive oil

¼ cup balsamic vinegar

2 teaspoons fresh chopped basil leaves, or 1 teaspoon dried *

Cook spaghetti according to package directions; drain and rinse
in cold water. Combine cooked spaghetti, cheese, tomatoes,
green onions, artichokes, and onion in a large bowl.

Place oil in a separate bowl; slowly whisk in vinegar to emul-
sify. Mix in basil. Pour oil mixture over spaghetti and vegetables,
and toss to combine. Refrigerate for 1 hour before serving.

Makes 4 servings

Nutrition information per serving: Calories: 342; Total fat: 18.8 g;
   Saturated fat: 4.6 g; Trans fat: 0 g; Cholesterol: 15.2 mg; Sodium: 237 mg;
   Total carbohydrates: 32.4 g; Fiber: 7.7 g; Sugars: 5.9 g; Protein: 14.4 g

Turkey Bolognese with Roasted Red Bell Pepper

1 pound whole-wheat pasta *

1 tablespoon olive oil

2 teaspoons minced garlic ~

½ cup diced red onion ~

2 teaspoons ground fennel seed ~

2 teaspoons dried sage, * or ½ tablespoon fresh chopped

1 teaspoon ground black pepper

1 pound ground turkey breast

1 25-ounce jar tomato sauce with vegetables (such as mushrooms or peppers; no added sugar or corn syrup) +

1 cup diced roasted red bell peppers

Cook pasta according to package directions. Meanwhile, heat oil in a large skillet over low heat. Add garlic, onion, fennel seed, sage, and black pepper. Cook, stirring occasionally, until onion is translucent. Increase heat slightly and add turkey. Stir constantly until meat is broken up into small pieces and no pink color remains. Stir in tomato sauce and bell peppers, and heat another 5 minutes, until hot. Serve sauce over the pasta.

Makes 4 to 6 servings

Nutrition information per serving: Calories: 514; Total fat: 13.1 g; Saturated fat: 2.6 g; Trans fat: 0 g; Cholesterol: 64.3 mg; Sodium: 664 mg; Total carbohydrates: 69.3 g; Fiber: 9.4 g; Sugars: 8.5 g; Protein: 26.2 g

▶Recipes to Improve Constipation Symptoms

Baked Tortilla Chips or Whole-Wheat Pita Chips

4 small whole-wheat pitas * or 8-inch corn tortillas,
cut into 8 wedges
Cooking spray
Mrs. Dash or other salt-free seasoning *

Preheat oven to 350°F. Lightly coat pita or tortilla wedges with cooking spray, and sprinkle with seasoning. Arrange on a baking sheet, and toast in oven for about 5 minutes, until crispy.

Makes 4 servings

Nutrition information per serving: Calories: 85; Total fat: 0.8 g; Saturated fat: 0.1 g; Trans fat: 0 g; Cholesterol: 0 mg; Sodium: 170 mg; Total carbohydrates: 17.6 g; Fiber: 2.4 g; Sugars: 0 g; Protein: 3.1 g

Barley Breakfast Cereal

1 cup low-fat milk + ■
½ cup quick-cooking barley *
1 tablespoon pure maple syrup
¼ teaspoon ground cinnamon
2 tablespoons chopped almonds or walnuts ~
2 tablespoons raisins

In a small pot, bring milk to a boil. Stir in remaining ingredients, and simmer over low heat for 10 minutes. Remove from heat, cover, and allow to sit for 5 minutes. Stir and serve.

Makes 2 servings

Nutrition information per serving—includes walnuts, versus almonds:
Calories: 233; Total fat: 7 g; Saturated fat: 1 g; Trans fat: 0 g; Cholesterol: 6 mg; Sodium: 61 mg; Total carbohydrates: 39 g; Fiber: 4 g; Sugars: 18 g; Protein: 9 g

Black Bean Dip with Tahini

Delicious and healthful served with raw vegetables and Whole-Wheat Pita Chips (see Index) or crackers made with no trans fats.

> 1 small bunch green onions, chopped (white part only) ~
> 1 tablespoon chopped fresh cilantro
> 2 tablespoons lemon juice +
> ½ cup tahini (sesame paste) *
> 1 15.5-ounce can black beans, drained and rinsed

In a serving bowl, combine green onions, cilantro, lemon juice, and tahini. Roughly mash beans in a food processor or blender. Add to bowl, and mix until blended.

Makes 16 servings

Nutrition information per serving: Calories: 69; Total fat: 4 g; Saturated fat: 1 g; Trans fat: 0 g; Cholesterol: 0 mg; Sodium: 87 mg; Total carbohydrates: 6 g; Fiber: 2 g; Sugars: 0 g; Protein: 3 g

Black-Eyed Pea Salad

1 15-ounce can low-sodium black-eyed peas, drained and rinsed
2 stalks celery, chopped fine
1 red bell pepper, chopped fine
4 green onions, sliced ~
2 carrots, peeled and grated
1/3 cup chopped cilantro
2 tablespoons Dijon mustard
1/3 cup low-fat Italian dressing ~

Place peas in a large bowl. Add celery, red bell pepper, green onions, and carrots. Toss cilantro. Set mixture aside. In a small bowl, combine the mustard and dressing. Pour over vegetable-pea mixture. Cover and marinate in refrigerator for 1 hour before serving.

Makes 4 servings

Nutrition information per serving: Calories: 202; Total fat: 5.6 g; Saturated fat: 0.9 g; Trans fat: 0 g; Cholesterol: 0 mg; Sodium: 318 mg; Total carbohydrates: 30.9 g; Fiber: 6.2 g; Sugars: 5 g; Protein: 9.8 g

Buckwheat Crepes

These crepes are even yummier stuffed with apple butter and sliced banana. Or use this recipe to create Raspberry and Cheese Blintzes (see Index) simply by adding filling. Buckwheat is also an excellent flour for people with diabetes, as it contains more fiber and protein than whole-wheat flour does.

    3 eggs, or equivalent amount of egg substitute
    2 tablespoons buckwheat flour
    1 tablespoon nonfat milk + ▦
    Cooking spray
    8 ounces sugar-free, fat-free fruit yogurt + ▦

Combine eggs, flour, milk, and 1 tablespoon of water in a blender or food processor. Cover and refrigerate for 3 hours or overnight. Batter should have the consistency of thin cream.

Coat a small (6-inch) skillet with cooking spray and place over high heat. When pan is hot, pour in about 1 tablespoon of batter. Tilt pan so that batter evenly coats the bottom. When small bubbles appear, use a spatula to flip the crepe, and cook for a few seconds on other side. Transfer crepe to a plate. Repeat with remaining batter.

Fold each crepe in half, and then fold in half again to make a quarter circle. Place three crepes on each of four serving plates, and spoon yogurt on top.

Makes 4 servings

Nutrition information per serving: Calories: 76; Total fat: 0.1 g; Saturated fat: 0 g; Trans fat: 0 g; Cholesterol: 1.8 mg; Sodium: 130 mg; Total carbohydrates: 11.1 g; Fiber: 0.8 g; Sugars: 6.4 g; Protein: 7.5 g

Cereal Cookies

Cooking spray

2 cups high-fiber, high-protein cereal (such as Kashi Just Friends or GoLean, or Weetabix flakes) *

¼ cup (1.5 ounces) raisins

½ cup chopped almonds, peanuts, or walnuts ~

½ teaspoon ground cinnamon

2 tablespoons ground flaxseed ~

3 egg whites

½ cup nonfat dry milk + ■

1 teaspoon vanilla extract

Preheat oven to 350°F. Coat a baking sheet with cooking spray.

In a large bowl, combine cereal, raisins, nuts, cinnamon, and flaxseed. Set aside. In another bowl, mix egg whites, dry milk, and vanilla until well blended. Pour egg white mixture into cereal mixture, and toss until cereal is well coated, forming cookie dough.

Place teaspoons of cookie dough a half inch apart on the baking sheet, pressing lightly on the top to form cookie shape. (Alternatively, to form into bars, divide mixture into six parts, wet hands lightly, and shape on pan.) Bake for 10 to 12 minutes, until lightly brown.

Makes about 26 servings (1 cookie per serving)

Nutrition information per serving: Calories: 42.8; Total fat: 1.7 g; Saturated fat: 0.1 g; Trans fat: 0 g; Cholesterol: 0.2 mg; Sodium: 21 mg; Total carbohydrates: 5.1 g; Fiber: 1.4 g; Sugars: 2.5 g; Protein: 2.7 g

Curried Butternut Squash, Garbanzo Beans, and Collard Greens

Look for green curry paste in the Asian section of your grocery store. Double your pleasure by serving this dish with Brown Basmati Rice Pilaf (see Index).

1 tablespoon safflower oil
½ cup diced red onion ~
3 cloves garlic, minced ~
1 medium butternut squash, peeled, seeded, and diced (about 2 cups)
1 cup canned low-sodium garbanzo beans
1½ cups skim milk + ■
1 cup nonfat dry milk + ■
½ cup low-sodium chicken or vegetable broth *
1½ teaspoons green curry paste *
1 tablespoon lime juice +
4 cups shredded collard greens (about 1 bunch), or 1 16-ounce package frozen chopped (thawed)
1 tablespoon coconut extract

Heat oil in a large skillet over medium heat. Add onion and garlic, and sauté gently until translucent. Add squash and beans, and stir to combine. In a small bowl, combine skim milk and dry milk; pour into pan. Add broth, curry paste, and lime juice, and stir to combine. Cover, reduce heat to low, and cook for 15 minutes. Add collard greens and coconut extract, and cook for 5 more minutes, or until squash is tender.

Makes 4 servings

Nutrition information per serving: Calories: 270; Total fat: 5.6 g; Saturated fat: 0.6 g; Trans fat: 0 g; Cholesterol: 3.4 mg; Sodium: 232 mg; Total carbohydrates: 43.5 g; Fiber: 6 g; Sugars: 17.4 g; Protein: 15 g

Falafel in Whole-Wheat Pita

You can also serve this no-fail falafel over a salad or by itself.

1 cup packed, flat Italian parsley leaves
1 small onion, quartered ~
2 15.5-ounce cans garbanzo beans, drained and rinsed
2 eggs
2 teaspoons dried cilantro, * or 4 teaspoons fresh chopped
2 tablespoons tahini (sesame paste) * ~
Olive or safflower oil
4 whole-wheat pitas *
8 lettuce leaves +
1 large tomato, sliced (about 2 slices per sandwich) +

In a food processor or blender, blend parsley and onion until smooth. Drain off liquid. Transfer to a small bowl and set aside. Place the beans in a food processor or blender, and blend until smooth. Add eggs one at a time, followed by onion-parsley mixture, cilantro, and tahini, blending until smooth.

Lightly coat a large skillet with oil, and heat over medium heat. Carefully place 1 tablespoon of batter at a time into the pan, and press with the back of the spoon to flatten slightly. Sauté until golden brown on the bottom, turn, and brown the other side.

(Instead of frying, you can bake these in a 375°F oven: Lightly coat a baking sheet with oil, and spoon the mixture onto the pan, again using the back of the spoon to flatten slightly. Bake for 15 to 20 minutes, or until set.)

Serve each patty in a whole-wheat pita with two lettuce leaves and tomato.

Makes 4 sandwiches

Nutrition information per serving: Calories: 620; Total fat: 19 g; Saturated fat: 3 g; Trans fat: 0 g; Cholesterol: 118 mg; Sodium: 1,107 mg; Total carbohydrates: 93 g; Fiber: 16 g; Sugars: 4 g; Protein: 24 g

Hearty Vegetable, Pearl Barley, and Kidney Bean Soup

½ cup pearl barley *
2 plum tomatoes, diced +
2 small carrots, peeled and diced
1 head fennel, diced
1 small zucchini, diced
1 red bell pepper, diced
4 ounces white mushrooms, washed and sliced
1 tablespoon canola oil
2 teaspoons chopped garlic ~
1 leek, diced (white and part of green)
1 10-ounce package frozen chopped kale, thawed and drained,
    or 1 cup fresh chopped
1 15.5-ounce can no-salt-added red kidney beans,
    drained and rinsed
1 48-ounce can low-sodium vegetable broth *
1 tablespoon dried basil, or 2 tablespoons fresh chopped *
1 tablespoon dried chives, or 2 tablespoons fresh chopped *
2 teaspoons dried oregano, or 4 teaspoons fresh chopped *

Rinse barley under cold water until water runs clear; drain and set aside. Combine tomatoes, carrots, fennel, zucchini, red bell pepper, and mushrooms; set aside.

Heat oil in a large skillet over medium heat. Add garlic and leek, and sauté for 2 minutes. Add the tomato-mushroom mixture, and continue to cook, stirring occasionally, for 5 more minutes. Stir in the kale, barley, beans, broth, basil, chives, and oregano. Lower heat, cover, and simmer for 40 to 50 minutes, until barley and vegetables are soft.

Makes about 8 servings

Nutrition information per serving: Calories: 174; Total fat: 3.1 g; Saturated
    fat: 0.2 g; Trans fat: 0 g; Cholesterol: 0 mg; Sodium: 498 mg; Total
    carbohydrates: 30.8 g; Fiber: 8 g; Sugars: 4 g; Protein: 7.4 g

Mango Salsa with Black Beans

This goes wonderfully with Poached Chicken Breast (see Index), or serve as a salad entree or over fish.

1 ripe mango, peeled and chopped (about 1½ cups)
¾ cup canned no-salt-added black beans, drained and rinsed
½ cup roasted red bell peppers, diced
1 small shallot, chopped fine (about 2 tablespoons) ~
1 small jalapeño pepper, seeded and minced
¼ cup chopped cilantro, minced
3 green onions, minced ~
½ teaspoon ground cumin *
¼ teaspoon cayenne pepper
3 tablespoons lime juice +
1 tablespoon olive oil
½ teaspoon kosher salt, optional

Place mango in a large bowl. Add black beans, bell peppers, and shallot. Stir in jalapeño, cilantro, and green onions. Add cumin, cayenne, lime juice, oil, and salt (optional), and mix well. Cover and refrigerate for at least 1 hour before serving. May be made a day ahead.

Makes about 16 servings

Nutrition information per serving: Calories: 41; Total fat: 1 g; Saturated fat: 0.1 g; Trans fat: 0 g; Cholesterol: 0 mg; Sodium: 107 mg; Total carbohydrates: 6.6 g; Fiber: 1.1 g; Sugars: 2.1 g; Protein: 1.2 g

Pumpkin and Quinoa Pudding

¾ cup pumpkin puree

1 teaspoon vanilla extract

2 tablespoons orange juice concentrate +

1 teaspoon pumpkin pie spice *

¼ cup pure maple syrup

1 cup low-fat plain yogurt + ■

1½ cups cooked quinoa

¼ cup walnuts, optional ~

Combine pumpkin, vanilla, orange juice concentrate, pumpkin pie spice, and maple syrup in a large bowl. Stir in yogurt, quinoa, and (optional) walnuts.

Makes 5 servings

Nutrition information per serving—including optional nuts: Calories: 201; Total fat: 6 g; Saturated fat: 1 g; Trans fat: 0 g; Cholesterol: 4 mg; Sodium: 41 mg; Total carbohydrates: 32 g; Fiber: 4 g; Sugars: 8 g; Protein: 5 g

Raspberry and Cheese Blintzes

A cheese filling plus Raspberry Sauce turns Buckwheat Crepes into Raspberry and Cheese Blintzes.

Buckwheat Crepes (See Index.)
Raspberry Sauce, thick version (See Index.)
1 cup fat-free ricotta cheese + ■
1 tablespoon ground cinnamon

For each of the twelve crepes, place 1 tablespoon sauce and 1 tablespoon ricotta in center of crepe, and fold in edges to overlap each other. Place three crepes, edges down, on each of four small plates, and sprinkle with cinnamon.

Makes 4 servings (3 filled crepes per serving)

Nutrition information per serving: Calories: 182; Total fat: 0.3 g; Saturated fat: 0.02 g; Trans fat: 0 g; Cholesterol: 11.8 mg; Sodium: 197 mg; Total carbohydrates: 29.1 g; Fiber: 2.5 g; Sugars: 13.1 g; Protein: 13.5 g

Raspberry Sauce

This recipe can be used to create a nice light sauce for desserts or adapted slightly to make a thicker sauce that is perfect for rolling inside crepes, such as with Raspberry and Cheese Blintzes. (See Index.)

1 10-ounce package frozen raspberries (no sugar added)

¼ cup orange juice +

½ teaspoon stevia powder

Optional for a thicker version: 2 teaspoons cornstarch

Combine raspberries and orange juice in a small pan; add stevia powder, and simmer until juices thicken slightly. Strain to remove seeds, and cool.

For a thicker sauce or filling, combine cornstarch with 1 tablespoon of water, and add to pan while ingredients are simmering. Simmer for 3 to 4 more minutes, stirring constantly. Strain to remove seeds, and cool.

Makes 3 servings

Nutrition information per serving: Calories: 51; Total fat: 0.1 g; Saturated fat: 0.01 g; Trans fat: 0 g; Cholesterol: 0 mg; Sodium: 0.7 mg; Total carbohydrates: 11.6 g; Fiber: 1.3 g; Sugars: 4.7 g; Protein: 1 g

Sesame Green Beans

1 pound fresh green beans, ends trimmed, or 1 12-ounce package
   frozen
1 tablespoon sesame oil
1 tablespoon sesame seeds ~

Cook beans in boiling water until slightly firm but not crisp;
drain. Heat oil in a large skillet over low heat. Add the beans,
and toss gently. Remove from heat. In a small pan, toast sesame
seeds over medium heat for about 2 to 3 minutes, stirring constantly to avoid burning. When you can smell the seeds, they are
almost done. Place the beans on a serving platter and sprinkle
with the toasted sesame seeds.

Makes 4 servings

Nutrition information per serving: Calories: 70; Total fat: 4.5 g; Saturated
fat: 0.5 g; Trans fat: 0 g; Cholesterol: 0 mg; Sodium: 4.2 mg; Total
carbohydrates: 7.1 g; Fiber: 4.3 g; Sugars: 2.7 g; Protein: 1.9 g

Spinach Salad

5 ounces baby spinach, washed and thoroughly dried
1 ripe pear, cored and diced
3 tablespoons crumbled Gorgonzola cheese + ▦
¼ cup dried cranberries *
4 tablespoons spiced walnuts ~
½ cup creamy cider dressing *

Place spinach in a serving bowl. Add pear, cheese, cranberries, and walnuts. Toss with dressing.

Makes 4 servings

Nutrition information per serving: Calories: 182; Total fat: 10 g; Saturated fat: 2 g; Trans fat: 0 g; Cholesterol: 5.8 mg; Sodium: 151 mg; Total carbohydrates: 22.1 g; Fiber: 4.7 g; Sugars: 11.4 g; Protein: 4.8 g

Strawberry, Banana, Yogurt, and Muesli Parfait

1½ cups plain low-fat yogurt + ■
½ teaspoon vanilla extract
½ teaspoon ground cinnamon
2 tablespoons pure maple syrup
1 cup muesli * ~
1 pint strawberries, stems removed and sliced
1 ripe banana, sliced

Combine yogurt, vanilla, cinnamon, and maple syrup.

For each serving, in a parfait glass or wineglass, layer ⅙ of the muesli, and then ⅓ each of the yogurt mixture, strawberries, and bananas, finishing with a layer of ⅙ of the muesli.

Makes 3 servings

Nutrition information per serving: Calories: 282; Total fat: 3 g; Saturated fat: 2 g; Trans fat: 0 g; Cholesterol: 10 mg; Sodium: 153 mg; Total carbohydrates: 58 g; Fiber: 6 g; Sugars: 35 g; Protein: 10 g

Tomato Salsa

Serve up this mouthwatering salsa with Baked Tortilla Chips or Whole-Wheat Pita Chips (see Index) and fresh vegetables.

2 large ripe tomatoes (about 1 pound), diced +
1 small jalapeño pepper, seeded and minced
2 cloves garlic, chopped ~
2 teaspoons dried cilantro, * or 4 teaspoons fresh chopped
16 medium pitted black olives, drained, rinsed, and chopped
2 tablespoons lime juice +

Place tomatoes in a serving bowl. Add jalapeño, garlic, and cilantro. Toss in olives and lime juice. Cover and refrigerate for 30 to 60 minutes before serving.

Makes 8 servings

Nutrition information per serving: Calories: 33; Total fat: 1.5 g; Saturated fat: 0 g; Trans fat: 0 g; Cholesterol: 0 mg; Sodium: 92 mg; Total carbohydrates: 4 g; Fiber: 0.5 g; Sugars: 1.6 g; Protein: 0.5 g

Trail Mix

1 cup old-fashioned oats *
Zest of 1 orange
1 cup sliced almonds ~
¼ cup honey
Cooking spray
½ cup (3 ounces) raisins
½ cup (3 ounces) peanuts ~
½ cup dried apricots cut into small pieces *

Preheat oven to 350°F. Combine oats, orange zest, and almonds. Spread mixture on an ungreased baking sheet; bake for 15 minutes. Remove from oven, but leave oven on.

Transfer toasted oat mixture to a large bowl, and stir in honey. Coat the baking sheet with cooking spray. Crumble the honey-oat mixture onto the sheet, and return to oven. Bake for about 10 minutes, or until golden. Allow mixture to cool, and then stir in raisins, peanuts, and apricots.

Makes 6 servings

Nutrition information per serving: Calories: 344; Total fat: 15 g; Saturated fat: 1 g; Trans fat: 0 g; Cholesterol: 0 mg; Sodium: 8 mg; Total carbohydrates: 45 g; Fiber: 6 g; Sugars: 22 g; Protein: 10 g

Zucchini Bread

Cooking spray
1 large ripe banana (or 2 small ones)
2 high-omega eggs
1 teaspoon vanilla extract
¼ cup canola oil
1 cup grated zucchini
½ cup oat bran *
¾ cup whole-wheat flour *
½ cup ground flaxseed ~
¾ cup (3 ounces) walnut pieces ~
½ cup (4 ounces) raisins
½ teaspoon salt
½ teaspoon baking powder
½ teaspoon baking soda
½ teaspoon ground cinnamon

Preheat oven to 350°F. Coat a 9″ × 5″ loaf pan or twelve 2½-inch muffin cups with cooking spray (or with a little oil and a dusting of flour).

In a blender or food processor, puree banana. Gradually add eggs and vanilla, and beat until smooth. Gradually add oil, and beat to combine. Pour the mixture into a large bowl, and stir in zucchini.

In a separate bowl, combine remaining ingredients. Add to the zucchini mixture, and blend thoroughly. Pour batter into prepared pan or muffin tin. Bake about 45 minutes for the loaf pan or 25 minutes for muffins. Bread is done when a toothpick inserted in center comes out dry.

Makes 12 servings

Nutrition information per serving: Calories: 209; Total fat: 13 g; Saturated fat: 1 g; Trans fat: 0 g; Cholesterol: 36 mg; Sodium: 188 mg; Total carbohydrates: 22 g; Fiber: 4 g; Sugars: 8 g; Protein: 5 g

▶Recipes to Improve GERD Symptoms

Maple Yogurt

Serve with banana pancakes or over fresh fruit; also luscious as a dip with sliced apples.

- 1 cup plain low-fat yogurt + ■
- 2 to 3 tablespoons pure maple syrup
- 1 teaspoon vanilla extract
- 1 teaspoon ground cinnamon

Combine all ingredients. Enjoy!

Makes 1 serving

Nutrition information per serving: Calories: 299; Total fat: 3 g; Saturated fat: 3 g; Trans fat: 0 g; Cholesterol: 20 mg; Sodium: 175 mg; Total carbohydrates: 52 g; Fiber: 1 g; Sugars: 46 g; Protein: 11 g

Strawberry Tofu "Ice Cream"

¼ 14-ounce package firm tofu
1 cup frozen strawberries (no sugar added)
½ teaspoon vanilla extract
1 tablespoon honey or pure maple syrup
¼ to ⅓ cup soy milk or low-fat milk + ▉
¼ cup muesli * ~

In a food processor or blender, combine tofu, strawberries, vanilla, and honey. Blend until smooth, adding just enough milk to achieve desired consistency. Pour mixture into a serving dish, and top with muesli.

Makes 1 serving

Nutrition information per serving: Calories: 321; Total fat: 8 g; Saturated fat: 1 g; Trans fat: 0 g; Cholesterol: 0 mg; Sodium: 94 mg; Total carbohydrates: 54 g; Fiber: 6g; Sugars: 31 g; Protein: 15 g

▶Recipes to Improve Dyspepsia Symptoms

Ginger Butternut Squash Soup

2 tablespoons olive oil

1 onion, diced ~

3 carrots, peeled and sliced

2 tablespoons peeled and chopped gingerroot

1 large butternut squash (about 4 to 5 pounds), peeled, seeded, and cut into 1- to 2-inch pieces

1 teaspoon ground cinnamon

1 48-ounce can low-sodium chicken or vegetable stock *

13 ounces 1% milk + ▪

1 teaspoon coconut extract

Salt and pepper to taste

Heat oil in large skillet over medium heat. Add onion, and sauté until translucent. Add carrots and gingerroot, and cook for 3 to 5 more minutes over medium to low heat. Stir in the squash, cinnamon, stock, milk, and coconut extract. Simmer over low heat for about 30 to 40 minutes, or until squash and carrots are soft. Remove from heat, allow to cool slightly; puree in a blender or food processor. Season with salt and pepper.

Makes 11 servings

Nutrition information per serving: Calories: 144; Total fat: 4 g; Saturated fat: 1 g; Trans fat: 0 g; Cholesterol: 2 mg; Sodium: 95 mg; Total carbohydrates: 25 g; Fiber: 6g; Sugars: 6 g; Protein: 6 g

Hummus

It's hard to beat this treat when served with fresh vegetables or with Baked Tortilla Chips or Whole-Wheat Pita Chips. (See Index.)

1 15.5-ounce can no-salt-added garbanzo beans, drained and rinsed
2 teaspoons ground cumin *
1 cup packed, flat Italian parsley leaves
5 tablespoons lemon juice +
2 cloves garlic ~
2 tablespoons tahini (sesame paste) *

Combine all ingredients in a blender or food processor; pulse until pureed.

Makes 7 servings

Nutrition information per serving: Calories: 138; Total fat: 4.1 g; Saturated fat: 0.5 g; Trans fat: 0 g; Cholesterol: 0 mg; Sodium: 15.5 mg; Total carbohydrates: 20.1 g; Fiber: 3.5 g; Sugars: 3.4 g; Protein: 6.7 g

Peach Yogurt Smoothie

You can use frozen, unthawed peaches in this recipe to create a "frozen yogurt" texture.

   ¾ cup fresh or frozen peaches (thawed)
   ½ cup plain low-fat yogurt + ■
   ½ teaspoon vanilla extract
   ¼ teaspoon ground cinnamon
   1 tablespoon orange juice concentrate +

Place all ingredients in a blender, and puree until smooth. To your health!

Makes 1 serving

Nutrition information per serving: Calories: 163; Total fat: 2 g; Saturated fat: 1 g; Trans fat: 0 g; Cholesterol: 10 mg; Sodium: 86 mg; Total carbohydrates: 29 g; Fiber: 3 g; Sugars: 15 g; Protein: 7 g

Recipes to Improve Celiac Sprue Symptoms

Always check all labeled products to be sure they are gluten free.

Almond-Crusted Baked Chicken Breast

¾ pound skinless, boneless chicken breast (organic if possible),
    visible fat trimmed
1 tablespoon Dijon mustard
1 cup almond meal or sliced almonds ground in a coffee grinder ~

Preheat oven to 350°F. Cover chicken breasts with plastic wrap, and pound to reduce thickness by half. Spread mustard on both sides of chicken, and dredge in almond meal. Place chicken on a baking sheet, and bake for about 20 minutes, or until meat is completely white when pierced.

Makes 2 servings

Nutrition information per serving: Calories: 575; Total fat: 40 g; Saturated fat: 6 g; Trans fat: 0 g; Cholesterol: 109 mg; Sodium: 578 mg; Total carbohydrates: 11 g; Fiber: 6 g; Sugars: 2 g; Protein: 46 g

Brown Basmati Rice with Ground Flax

1 tablespoon canola oil
½ small onion, diced ~
1 small red bell pepper, diced
½ cup brown basmati rice
1½ cups chicken or vegetable stock *
1 bay leaf
¼ cup ground flaxseed ~
1 bunch green onions, sliced (white and part of green part) ~

Heat oil in a large skillet over low heat. Add onion and bell pepper, and sauté until soft. Stir in rice, stock, and bay leaf. Cover skillet, and simmer for about 45 minutes. Remove from heat, and allow to sit covered for 5 more minutes. Before serving, remove bay leaf, and stir in flaxseed and green onions.

Makes 2 servings

Nutrition information per serving: Calories: 183; Total fat: 9 g; Saturated fat: 1 g; Trans fat: 0 g; Cholesterol: 2 mg; Sodium: 384 mg; Total carbohydrates: 24 g; Fiber: 5 g; Sugars: 2 g; Protein: 5 g

Fruit Soup

1 pint strawberries, stemmed
1 mango, peeled and cut into small pieces
1 large banana, cut into small pieces
½ cantaloupe, cut into small pieces
1 cup orange juice +

Place all fruits and orange juice in a blender or food processor; blend until smooth. Chill before serving.

Makes 5 servings

Nutrition information per serving: Calories: 119; Total fat: 1 g; Saturated fat: 0 g; Trans fat: 0 g; Cholesterol: 0 mg; Sodium: 15 mg; Total carbohydrates: 29 g; Fiber: 3 g; Sugars: 17 g; Protein: 1 g

Green Pea Soup

This soup can be served hot or cold.

2 ripe avocados, peeled, pitted, and cut into pieces
¼ cup lemon juice +
20 to 24 ounces low-sodium chicken broth *
1 16-ounce package frozen green peas, thawed
1 teaspoon ground cumin *
½ teaspoon salt

Toss avocado pieces with lemon juice and set aside. In a sauce-pan, bring broth and peas to a boil. Remove from heat; drain broth and reserve. Place peas and avocado-lemon mixture in a blender or food processor, and puree until smooth. Gradually add the reserved broth until soup is of desired consistency. Stir in cumin and salt.

Makes about 6 servings

Nutrition information per serving: Calories: 177; Total fat: 11 g; Saturated fat: 2 g; Trans fat: 0 g; Cholesterol: 0 mg; Sodium: 393 mg; Total carbohydrates: 18 g; Fiber: 8 g; Sugars: 6 g; Protein: 7 g

Mediterranean Tuna Salad

3 ounces baby arugula, washed and thoroughly dried
½ cup balsamic vinaigrette *
1 6-ounce can light tuna packed in water, drained
1 6-ounce jar marinated artichoke hearts (no hydrogenated oil),
   drained and cut in half
½ 12-ounce jar roasted sweet red bell peppers, drained
3 to 4 ounces oil-cured or kalamata olives
1 ripe avocado, peeled, pitted, and diced

Toss the arugula with vinaigrette, and divide between two salad
bowls. Spoon the tuna down the center of each bowl, followed by
artichoke, bell peppers, olives, and avocado.

Makes 2 servings

Nutrition information per serving: Calories: 726; Total fat: 50 g; Saturated
   fat: 6 g; Trans fat: 0 g; Cholesterol: 53 mg; Sodium: 2,710 mg; Total
   carbohydrates: 41 g; Fiber: 12 g; Sugars: 12 g; Protein: 32 g

Roasted Beet, Baby Spinach, and Goat Cheese Salad

12 to 16 ounces fresh beets, root ends and stems removed
½ cup Walnut Vinaigrette, divided (See Index.)
3 ounces baby spinach, washed and thoroughly dried
2 to 3 ounces pasteurized goat cheese, crumbled + ■
2 ounces walnuts, chopped ~

Preheat oven to 350°F. Place beets in a baking dish, cover with foil, and bake until a fork easily pierces each, about 30 to 40 minutes, depending on size of beets.

Allow beets to cool, and then peel and dice. Marinate the beets for 15 minutes in ¼ cup Walnut Vinaigrette. Toss the spinach with remaining Walnut Vinaigrette; add the beets and cheese. Top with walnuts.

Makes 2 servings

Nutrition information per serving: Calories: 469; Total fat: 36 g; Saturated fat: 10 g; Trans fat: 0 g; Cholesterol: 28 mg; Sodium: 372 mg; Total carbohydrates: 25 g; Fiber: 8 g; Sugars: 15 g; Protein: 16 g

Sweet Potato Pudding

Cooking spray

1⅓ cups mashed, cooked sweet potato

½ cup sugar

2 teaspoons ground cinnamon

2 teaspoons grated orange rind

1 teaspoon salt (omit if on a low-sodium diet)

1 teaspoon ground gingerroot *

½ teaspoon ground cloves *

⅓ cup egg substitute *

16 ounces evaporated skim milk + ▪

Preheat oven to 375°F. Coat a 2-quart casserole dish with cooking spray.

In a large bowl, combine sweet potato, sugar, cinnamon, orange rind, salt, gingerroot, cloves, and egg substitute. Beat with an electric mixer at medium speed until smooth. Add milk; mix well. Pour mixture into the casserole dish, and bake for 1 hour, or until a knife inserted near the center comes out clean. (For individual servings, pour ⅔ cup of the potato mixture into each of four custard cups. Bake for 40 minutes, or until a knife inserted near the center comes out clean.) Allow pudding to cool. Cover and refrigerate for 2 hours before serving.

Makes 4 servings

Nutrition information per serving: Calories: 304; Total fat: 1.3 g; Saturated fat: 0.4 g; Trans fat: 0 g; Cholesterol: 5.3 mg; Sodium: 828 mg; Total carbohydrates: 60.5 g; Fiber: 2.3 g; Sugars: 44.1 g; Protein: 13.9 g

Tilapia Tapenade

1 pound boneless tilapia fillets
Salt and pepper
2 tablespoons olive oil
3 cloves garlic, sliced ~
1 red bell pepper, seeded and julienned
2 tablespoons capers
1 6-ounce jar marinated artichoke hearts, undrained (Marinade
  should not contain hydrogenated oils.)
4 to 6 ounces quality pitted olives (niçoise, gaeta, country mix)
1 14.5-ounce can diced tomatoes (no sugar added), undrained +
2 tablespoons lemon juice +
4 large basil leaves, chopped

Preheat oven to 350°F. Sprinkle tilapia with salt and pepper. Heat oil in a large sauté pan. Add tilapia, and cook for 2 to 3 minutes on each side, until color turns from opaque to white. Transfer fillets to an ovenproof dish, and place in oven to finish cooking and keep warm while you prepare the sauce.

Place garlic in pan, and sauté until translucent. Add red bell pepper, capers, artichoke hearts with marinade, olives, tomatoes, lemon juice, and basil. Lower heat and simmer for 5 minutes. Season with salt and pepper.

Arrange fish on a serving plate, and spoon sauce on top.

Makes 2 servings

Nutrition information per serving: Calories: 487; Total fat: 28 g; Saturated fat: 3 g; Trans fat: 0 g; Cholesterol: 91 mg; Sodium: 1,668 mg; Total carbohydrates: 22 g; Fiber: 5 g; Sugars: 6 g; Protein: 42 g

Tofu Chili

Do your taste buds a favor by pairing this chili with Brown Basmati Rice with Ground Flax (see Index).

    1 14-ounce package firm tofu, frozen and thawed
    2 tablespoons canola oil
    1 small onion, diced ~
    2 cloves garlic, sliced ~
    1 green bell pepper, seeded and diced
    2 teaspoons ground cumin *
    2 teaspoons chili powder *
    1 teaspoon dried cilantro *
    1 tablespoon Worcestershire sauce *
    1 28-ounce can diced tomatoes (no sugar added), undrained +
    1 29-ounce can red kidney beans, drained and rinsed
    1 ripe avocado, peeled and pitted, cut into ½-inch pieces

Drain liquid from tofu, and crumble to resemble ground meat; set aside. Heat oil in a large skillet over medium heat. Add onion, garlic, and bell pepper, and sauté until onion is translucent. Stir in cumin, chili powder, cilantro, Worcestershire sauce, tomatoes, and beans. Reduce heat to low, and simmer for 20 minutes. Add the tofu, and simmer for 20 minutes more. Fold avocado in before serving.

Makes 6 servings

Nutrition information per serving: Calories: 358; Total fat: 14 g; Saturated fat: 2 g; Trans fat: 0 g; Cholesterol: 0 mg; Sodium: 352 mg; Total carbohydrates: 42 g; Fiber: 17 g; Sugars: 7 g; Protein: 18 g

Tofu Tomato Sauce

Enjoy this flavorful sauce over whole-wheat pasta or Barilla Plus pasta, which contains added protein, fiber, and omega-3.

3 tablespoons olive oil

8 cloves garlic, sliced ~

2 28-ounce cans ground peeled tomatoes (organic if possible— nothing added), undrained +

1 tablespoon dried oregano *

1 14-ounce package firm tofu, frozen and thawed

2 tablespoons fresh basil, chopped

Heat oil in a large skillet over low heat. Add garlic, and sauté until translucent. Add tomatoes and oregano. Simmer for 40 minutes, stirring occasionally. Remove any "foam" that forms on the top.

Crumble tofu, and add to sauce. Continue to simmer for 20 more minutes. Remove from heat, and stir in basil. For a smoother sauce, puree in a blender or food processor.

Makes 12 servings

Nutrition information per serving: Calories: 83; Total fat: 5 g; Saturated fat: 1 g; Trans fat: 0 g; Cholesterol: 0 g; Sodium: 86 mg; Total carbohydrates: 6 g; Fiber: 1 g; Sugars: 3 g; Protein: 5 g

Vegetable Dip

Serve with Baked Tortilla Chips or Whole-Wheat Pita Chips (see Index), fresh vegetables, or both.

1 8-ounce package low-fat cream cheese, softened + ▓
½ cup nonfat sour cream + ▓
1 tablespoon dried chives, * or 2 tablespoons fresh chopped
2 teaspoons prepared horseradish
1 teaspoon Worcestershire sauce *
1 teaspoon Mrs. Dash or other salt-free seasoning *
2 teaspoons hot sauce
1 teaspoon dry mustard
1 small bunch green onions, chopped (white and part of
   green portion) ~

Combine all ingredients in a serving bowl. Cover and refrigerate for 1 hour to allow flavors to blend before serving.

Makes 6 servings

Nutrition information per serving: Calories: 116; Total fat: 7 g; Saturated fat: 4 g; Trans fat: 0 g; Cholesterol: 23 mg; Sodium: 149 mg; Total carbohydrates: 7 g; Fiber: 1 g; Sugars: 2 g; Protein: 5 g

Walnut Vinaigrette

¼ cup orange juice +
2 tablespoons cider vinegar
1 teaspoon salt
½ cup walnut oil ~

Place orange juice, vinegar, and salt in a blender. Blend until smooth, slowly drizzling in oil. Cover and refrigerate.

Makes 6 servings

Nutrition information per serving: Calories: 83; Total fat: 9 g; Saturated fat: 1 g; Trans fat: 0 g; Cholesterol: 0 mg; Sodium: 194 mg; Total carbohydrates: 1 g; Fiber: 0 g; Sugars: 1 g; Protein: 0 g

Zesty Pumpkin Custards

2 tablespoons sugar

1 tablespoon honey

¾ teaspoon ground cinnamon

½ teaspoon ground allspice *

1 egg

6 ounces evaporated skim milk + ▪

8 ounces canned cooked pumpkin

¼ cup reduced-calorie frozen whipped topping, thawed * ▪

Preheat oven to 325°F. Combine sugar, honey, cinnamon, allspice, egg, milk, and pumpkin in a large bowl. Using an electric mixer, beat at low speed until smooth. Spoon ½ cup of the mixture into each of four 6-ounce ramekins or custard cups. Place the ramekins in a 9-inch square baking pan; add hot water to the pan to a depth of 1 inch. Bake for 1 hour, or until set. Remove ramekins from pan and allow to cool. Top each serving with 1 tablespoon whipped topping.

Makes 4 servings

Nutrition information per serving: Calories: 124; Total fat: 1.9 g; Saturated fat: 0.5 g; Trans fat: 0 g; Cholesterol: 48.4 mg; Sodium: 73.4 mg; Total carbohydrates: 21.6 g; Fiber: 1.9 g; Sugars: 18.4 g; Protein: 5.6 g

▶Recipes to Improve Multiple Conditions

Baked Chicken with Brown Basmati Rice

Improves diarrhea, dyspepsia, and GERD

1 quartered chicken (4 to 4½ pounds)
1 10-ounce package frozen chopped broccoli, thawed
1 cup brown basmati rice
1½ cups low-sodium chicken broth *
2 bay leaves
2 cups low-sugar, low-sodium tomato sauce +

Preheat oven to 350°F. Remove skin and any visible fat from chicken. Squeeze excess water from broccoli. Rinse rice.

In a saucepan, bring broth and bay leaves to a boil over medium heat. Lower heat; stir in tomato sauce, and heat through. Place rice and broccoli in a baking pan, and stir to combine. Pour sauce over rice mixture, removing bay leaves. Place chicken on top, meat side down. Cover tightly with aluminum foil or lid, and bake for 75 minutes.

Remove foil (being careful to avoid steam) and check for doneness: the rice should be soft, and chicken meat should be white. If necessary, recover tightly and cook for an additional 10 to 15 minutes.

Makes 4 servings

Nutrition information per serving: Calories: 492; Total fat: 8.5 g; Saturated fat: 1.9 g; Trans fat: 0 g; Cholesterol: 144.6 mg; Sodium: 183.4 mg; Total carbohydrates: 44.8 g; Fiber: 5.5 g; Sugars: 1 g; Protein: 61.4 g

Corn-Crusted Cod

Improves diarrhea and dyspepsia

You can substitute halibut, tilapia, or haddock for the cod. This dish is all the more taste tempting served alongside Mango Salsa with Black Beans (see Index).

Cooking spray
1 cup polenta (roughly ground cornmeal)
1 teaspoon ground cumin *
2 teaspoons chopped fresh parsley, or 1 teaspoon dried *
1 teaspoon ground white pepper
½ teaspoon paprika
1 cup nonfat buttermilk (or add 1 tablespoon vinegar to 1 cup nonfat milk to create buttermilk) ▪
4 4-ounce cod fillets

Preheat oven to 375°F. Generously coat a baking sheet with cooking spray.

In a large bowl, combine polenta with cumin, parsley, pepper, and paprika. Pour buttermilk into another large bowl. Dip each fillet into the buttermilk, allowing excess to drain off, and then coat on all sides with polenta mixture. Arrange the fillets on the baking sheet, and bake for about 10 to 15 minutes, until outside is golden brown and firm to the touch; fish should flake apart easily, and flesh should be white.

Makes 4 servings

Nutrition information per serving: Calories: 325; Total fat: 5.1 g; Saturated fat: 1.6 g; Trans fat: 0 g; Cholesterol: 69 mg; Sodium: 562 mg; Total carbohydrates: 34.7 g; Fiber: 3.1 g; Sugars: 5 g; Protein: 33.7 g

Fruit Smoothie

Improves constipation, GERD, and dyspepsia

This is a terrific way to use bananas that are getting too ripe. You can always cut ripe bananas in half and freeze them ahead of time; thaw when you're ready to make another smoothie.

   ¾ cup plain nonfat yogurt + ■
   ½ cup frozen blueberries
   ½ ripe banana
   1 teaspoon ground cinnamon
   1 teaspoon vanilla extract
   1 tablespoon ground flaxseed ~

Place all ingredients in a blender or food processor, and blend to combine.

Makes 1 serving

Nutrition information per serving: Calories: 221; Total fat: 3.5 g; Saturated fat: 0.3 g; Trans fat: 0 g; Cholesterol: 3.7 mg; Sodium: 106 mg; Total carbohydrates: 41.4 g; Fiber: 6.4 g; Sugars: 23.5 g; Protein: 10.3 g

Lentil Soup

Improves celiac sprue and dyspepsia

High in protein, fiber, folacin, phosphorus, potassium, iron, vitamin A, and beta-carotene.

½ cup wild brown rice
3 tablespoons canola oil
1 cup diced carrots
1 cup diced onion ~
1 cup diced fennel +
3 cloves garlic, chopped ~
1½ cups lentils
2 teaspoons dried thyme *
2 teaspoons ground cumin *
2 bay leaves
2 32-ounce containers chicken or vegetable broth *

Rinse and drain rice. Over medium heat, heat oil in a large sauce pot. Add carrots, onion, fennel, and garlic, and sauté until translucent. Stir in lentils, rice, thyme, cumin, bay leaves, and broth.

Bring to a boil; lower heat, cover, and simmer for about 1 hour, or until rice is cooked. Remove bay leaves before serving.

Makes 6 servings

Nutrition information per serving: Calories: 343; Total fat: 10 g; Saturated fat: 1 g; Trans fat: 0 g; Cholesterol: 0 mg; Sodium: 269 mg; Total carbohydrates: 48 g; Fiber: 18 g; Sugars: 3 g; Protein: 16 g

Poached Chicken Breast

Improves diarrhea and celiac sprue

This versatile dish may be served cold as a fancy salad entree by dicing the cooked meat, mixing it into Mango Salsa with Black Beans (see Index), and adding arugula; or serve it hot alongside Mango Salsa with Black Beans.

    2 cups low-sodium chicken broth *
    2 bay leaves
    4 to 6 sprigs fresh thyme, or 2 teaspoons dried *
    4 skinless, boneless chicken breast halves

In a large saucepan, combine broth, bay leaves, and thyme, and bring to a simmer over low heat. Remove any visible fat from chicken. Add chicken to broth, and continue to simmer for about 15 to 18 minutes, until meat is completely white. Remove pan from heat, and allow contents to cool. Remove chicken from poaching liquid and serve, or refrigerate and serve cold.

Makes 4 servings

Nutrition information per serving: Calories: 196; Total fat: 4.1 g; Saturated fat: 1.1 g; Trans fat: 0 g; Cholesterol: 98.9 mg; Sodium: 384 mg; Total carbohydrates: 0.7 g; Fiber: 0.1 g; Sugars: 0.5 g; Protein: 36.2 g

Poached Salmon Sandwich

Improves diarrhea and dyspepsia

2 bay leaves
2 cloves garlic, sliced ~
1 teaspoon dried thyme leaves, * or 4 sprigs fresh
4 3-ounce skinless, boneless salmon fillets
1 tablespoon low-fat or fat-free mayonnaise *
2 teaspoons Dijon mustard
4 whole-wheat rolls *
1 ripe avocado, peeled and pitted, cut into 8 wedges
4 tomato slices +
1 bunch arugula, washed and dried

Place bay leaves, garlic, and thyme in a large skillet. Add salmon, and cover contents with water. Bring to a simmer and cook until salmon is opaque throughout. Remove salmon, and allow fillets to cool. Combine mayonnaise and mustard, and set aside.

To assemble sandwiches: Spread mustard-mayonnaise mixture on inside of each roll. Add one salmon fillet, two slices of avocado, and one slice of tomato, and top with arugula. Close up roll.

Makes 4 servings

Nutrition information per serving—based on low-fat mayonnaise:
Calories: 434; Total fat: 20 g; Saturated fat: 3.4 g; Trans fat: 0 g; Cholesterol: 60.6 mg; Sodium: 584 mg; Total carbohydrates: 40.7 g; Fiber: 8.7 g; Sugars: 7.3 g; Protein: 26.1 g

Raspberry-Peach Jell-O Terrine

Improves constipation and GERD

This recipe uses Greek yogurt, which has a thicker consistency than regular yogurt. If you can't find it at your grocery store, you can substitute regular nonfat plain yogurt or even fat-free sour cream.

> 8 arrowroot cookies
> 1 small package sugar-free raspberry Jell-O ~
> 1 cup fat-free plain Greek yogurt or regular fat-free plain yogurt + ■
> 1 15-ounce can light sliced peaches, drained and chopped

Break cookies into medium-size pieces, and place in freezer for 20 minutes (this helps to keep them from getting too soggy in the Jell-O). Bring 1 cup of water to a boil in a saucepan. Remove pan from heat, pour in Jell-O, and stir to dissolve completely. Add ½ cup of cold water and yogurt; mix completely. Add peaches. Pour mixture into a 1-quart container. Refrigerate for 10 minutes to allow Jell-O to thicken and begin to set. Mix in the cold cookie pieces, and refrigerate for about 1 more hour, until completely set.

Makes 4 servings

Nutrition information per serving: Calories: 129; Total fat: 0.7 g; Saturated fat: 0.2 g; Trans fat: 0 g; Cholesterol: 1.2 mg; Sodium: 143 mg; Total carbohydrates: 28.6 g; Fiber: 1.4 g; Sugars: 3.2 g; Protein: 4.6 g

Salmon Salad

Improves celiac sprue and diarrhea

Serve mounded on a bed of mixed greens, or in a whole-wheat pita pocket or whole-wheat wrap with lettuce and tomato.

    1 7.5-ounce can pink salmon, drained and flaked
    1 6-ounce jar marinated artichoke hearts, drained and chopped
    1 cup cooked broccoli, chopped
    2 tablespoons lemon juice +
    2 tablespoons olive oil
    ½ teaspoon dried thyme *
    ½ teaspoon dried oregano *
    ½ teaspoon onion powder *
    2 tablespoons chopped capers

Combine salmon, artichoke, broccoli, lemon juice, oil, thyme, oregano, onion powder, and capers. Eat up!

Makes 2 servings

Nutrition information per serving: Calories: 376; Total fat: 24 g; Saturated fat: 3 g; Trans fat: 0 g; Cholesterol: 87 mg; Sodium: 1,031 mg; Total carbohydrates: 17 g; Fiber: 6 g; Sugars: 2 g; Protein: 30 g

Turkey Meat Loaf

Improves dyspepsia and GERD

1 small red onion, diced fine +
1 small red bell pepper, diced fine
1 cup grated carrot
1 teaspoon fresh thyme leaves, or ½ teaspoon dried *
1 teaspoon fresh sage, or ½ teaspoon dried *
1 tablespoon olive oil
½ cup plain bread crumbs *
1 teaspoon ground black pepper
1 egg
1 pound ground turkey breast meat *

Preheat oven to 350°F. Coat a loaf pan with cooking spray.

Combine onion and red bell pepper with carrot. Chop thyme and sage, and add to vegetables. Heat oil in a large skillet over medium heat. Add vegetables and cook, stirring constantly, until onion is soft and transparent. Remove pan from heat, and allow contents to cool. Add bread crumbs, black pepper, and egg to vegetables; mix to combine. Add ground turkey, and mix well. Press mixture into the loaf pan. Bake for about 1 hour, or until juices run clear and meat is no longer pink.

Makes 4 servings

Nutrition information per serving: Calories: 309; Total fat: 15.8 g; Saturated fat: 4.5 g; Trans fat: 0 g; Cholesterol: 142.9 mg; Sodium: 280 mg; Total carbohydrates: 16.5 g; Fiber: 2.4; Sugars: 3.9 g; Protein: 24.6 g

Nutritious Recipes for People with Diabetes

The following recipes can be used to create menus that fit into your calorie and fat-gram targets for your snacks, light meal, or main meal of the day. All of the main dishes contain fewer than 300 calories and 10 grams of fat per serving.

Asian-Style Chicken-Peanut Pasta

1 teaspoon sugar

1 teaspoon cornstarch

1 teaspoon peeled, minced gingerroot

2 tablespoons plus 1 teaspoon low-sodium soy sauce

1 teaspoon white vinegar +

⅛ teaspoon hot sauce

2 to 3 cloves garlic, minced ~

½ pound skinless, boneless chicken breast, cut into thin strips

1 teaspoon vegetable oil

1 cup minced green onions

1 cup fresh snow peas, halved

2½ cups hot cooked fusilli (corkscrew pasta), cooked without
   salt or fat *

1 teaspoon dark sesame oil

¼ cup unsalted dry-roasted peanuts ~

Combine sugar, cornstarch, gingerroot, the 2 tablespoons soy sauce, vinegar, hot sauce, garlic, and ½ cup of water in a large bowl; stir well. Add chicken, tossing gently to coat. Cover and refrigerate for 1 hour.

Remove chicken from marinade (reserve). Heat oil in a large skillet over medium-high heat. Add the chicken, and stir-fry for about 5 minutes, until meat is cooked through. Add reserved marinade, green onions, and peas; stir-fry 2 minutes, or until slightly thickened. Remove from heat. Combine fusilli, sesame oil, and remaining 1 teaspoon soy sauce in a large bowl; toss gently to coat pasta. Add chicken mixture, and top with peanuts, tossing gently.

Makes 4 servings

Nutrition information per serving: Calories: 298; Total fat: 8.4 g; Saturated fat: 1.2 g; Trans fat: 0 g; Cholesterol: 32.5 mg; Sodium: 86.4 mg; Total carbohydrates: 34.1 g; Fiber: 3.8 g; Sugars: 3.4 g; Protein: 20.7 g

Chicken Thighs with Roasted Apples and Garlic

4½ cups chopped, peeled Braeburn apples (about 1½ pounds)
1 teaspoon chopped fresh sage
½ teaspoon ground cinnamon *
½ teaspoon ground nutmeg *
4 cloves garlic, chopped ~
½ teaspoon salt (omit if on a low-sodium diet)
8 chicken thighs (about 2 pounds), skinned
¼ teaspoon ground black pepper

Preheat oven to 475°F. Coat a jelly roll pan with cooking spray.

Combine apples, sage, cinnamon, nutmeg, and garlic in a large bowl. Add ¼ teaspoon of the salt, and mix well. Spread the apple mixture on the jelly roll pan. Sprinkle the chicken with the remaining ¼ teaspoon salt and the pepper, and arrange thighs on top of the apple mixture. Bake for 25 minutes, or until chicken is cooked through and apple pieces are tender.

Remove chicken from pan; keep warm. Transfer apple mixture to a bowl, and partially mash with a potato masher. Serve with chicken.

Makes 4 servings

Nutrition information per serving: Calories: 183; Total fat: 3.6 g; Saturated fat: 0.9 g; Trans fat: 0.1 g; Cholesterol: 68.1 mg; Sodium: 361 mg; Total carbohydrates: 22.2 g; Fiber: 2.5 g; Sugars: 17.1 g; Protein: 16.7 g

Chilled Couscous Salad

1½ cups no-salt-added chicken broth *
½ cup couscous *
½ cup seeded, chopped, unpeeled tomato +
¾ cup chopped red bell pepper
⅓ cup chopped celery
⅓ cup seeded, chopped, unpeeled cucumber
¼ cup chopped green onions
¼ cup chopped fresh parsley
2 tablespoons balsamic vinegar +
1 tablespoon olive oil
1 tablespoon Dijon mustard
½ teaspoon grated lemon zest
¼ teaspoon ground black pepper

In a medium saucepan, bring broth to a boil over high heat. Stir in couscous. Remove from heat, cover, and allow to stand for 5 minutes. Fluff with a fork, and allow to cool uncovered for 10 minutes. Combine cooked couscous, tomato, bell pepper, celery, cucumber, green onions, and parsley in a large bowl, and toss gently.

In a small bowl, combine vinegar, oil, mustard, lemon zest, and black pepper. Stir with a whisk. Add to couscous mixture, and toss to coat. Serve chilled or at room temperature.

Makes 4 servings

Nutrition information per serving: Calories: 154; Total fat: 4.4 g; Saturated fat: 0.7 g; Trans fat: 0 g; Cholesterol: 0 mg; Sodium: 85.2 mg; Total carbohydrates: 23.2 g; Fiber: 2.6 g; Sugars: 3.6 g; Protein: 5.6 g

Chilled Multi-Melon Summertime Soup

3 cups cubed honeydew melon
3 cups cubed cantaloupe
¼ cup vodka
¼ cup firmly packed brown sugar
4 teaspoons fresh lime juice
¾ cup sliced strawberries

In a blender or food processor, process honeydew until smooth; pour into a bowl. Place cantaloupe in blender, and process until smooth; pour into another bowl. To each bowl of pureed melon, add 2 tablespoons of the vodka, 2 tablespoons of the brown sugar, and 2 teaspoons of the lime juice; stir well. Cover and refrigerate. Place strawberries in blender; process until smooth. Pour into a bowl; cover and chill.

To serve, evenly divide the cantaloupe mixture among four individual bowls. Pour ½ cup of the honeydew mixture into the center of each. Dollop each serving with 2 tablespoons of the pureed strawberries, and swirl decoratively with a wooden pick.

Makes 4 servings

Nutrition information per serving: Calories: 188; Total fat: 0.5 g; Saturated fat: 0.1 g; Trans fat: 0 g; Cholesterol: 0 mg; Sodium: 49.5 mg; Total carbohydrates: 40 g; Fiber: 2.9 g; Sugars: 36.2 g; Protein: 2.1 g

Fresh Vegetable Mélange

1½ teaspoons vegetable oil
1½ cups sliced onion, separated into rings
1 cup red bell pepper strips
2 cloves garlic, minced ~
1¾ cups sliced yellow squash
1¾ cups sliced zucchini
1 cup chopped, unpeeled plum tomatoes +
1 tablespoon julienned fresh basil
½ teaspoon lemon pepper
¼ teaspoon salt (omit if on a low-sodium diet)
1 tablespoon grated Parmesan cheese ■

Heat oil in a large nonstick skillet over medium-high heat. Add onion, bell pepper, and garlic; stir-fry for 2 minutes. Add squash and zucchini; stir-fry for 3 more minutes, or until the vegetables are crisp-tender. Add tomatoes, basil, lemon pepper, and salt; cook for 1 minute, or until thoroughly heated. Sprinkle with cheese before serving.

Makes 4 servings

Nutrition information per serving: Calories: 70.2; Total fat: 2.4 g; Saturated fat: 0.4 g; Trans fat: 0 g; Cholesterol: 1.1 mg; Sodium: 175 mg; Total carbohydrates: 10.9 g; Fiber: 2.9 g; Sugars: 6 g; Protein: 2.9 g

Ginger-Infused Beef and Pineapple Stir-Fry

½ pound lean flank steak

1 tablespoon peeled, minced gingerroot

2 teaspoons sugar

1½ tablespoons low-sodium soy sauce

1½ tablespoons sherry +

2 cloves garlic, minced ~

2 teaspoons cornstarch

4 teaspoons rice vinegar +

Cooking spray

2 teaspoons dark sesame oil

1½ cups cubed fresh pineapple

½ cup diagonally sliced (3-inch) green onions

½ cup thinly sliced fresh mushrooms

½ cup fresh snow peas (¼ pound)

½ cup julienned (3-inch) red bell pepper

4 cups hot cooked somen noodles or angel hair pasta, cooked
   without salt or fat *

Trim fat from steak. Cut steak lengthwise with the grain into
¼-inch-thick slices, and then cut these slices in half crosswise.
Combine steak, gingerroot, sugar, soy sauce, sherry, and garlic
in a large zip-top heavy-duty plastic bag. Seal bag, and marinate
steak in refrigerator for 2 hours, turning the bag occasionally.
Remove steak from bag, and discard the marinade.

In a small bowl, combine cornstarch and vinegar. Stir well
and set aside. Coat a large nonstick skillet with cooking spray.
Pour oil into pan, and heat over medium-high heat until hot. Add
the steak, and stir-fry for 4 minutes. Add the cornstarch mixture, pineapple, green onions, mushrooms, peas, and bell pepper
to the skillet; stir-fry for 3 minutes, or until vegetables are crisp-
tender. Serve over noodles.

Makes 4 servings

Nutrition information per serving: Calories: 391; Total fat: 2.6 g; Saturated
   fat: 0.3 g; Trans fat: 0 g; Cholesterol: 0 mg; Sodium: 229 mg; Total
   carbohydrates: 54.9 g; Fiber: 3.1 g; Sugars: 14.2 g; Protein: 1.4 g

Gorgonzola Bruschetta with Crisp Apple Slices

⅓ cup crumbled Gorgonzola or other type of blue cheese ■
1½ teaspoons butter, softened ■
1 teaspoon brandy or cognac
¼ teaspoon ground black pepper
4 1-inch-thick diagonal slices French bread (about 1 ounce each) *
2 cloves garlic, halved ~
1 medium Granny Smith apple, cut into 8 wedges

Coat a grill or grill pan with cooking spray. Combine the cheese, butter, brandy, and pepper in a small bowl, stirring until well blended. Arrange the bread on the grill, and cook for 2 minutes on each side, or until slightly brown. Remove bread, and rub the cut sides of the garlic over one side of each bread slice. Spread 2 teaspoons of the cheese mixture on top of each. Serve with two apple wedges apiece.

Makes 4 servings

Nutrition information per serving: Calories: 264; Total fat: 5.9 g; Saturated fat: 3.2 g; Trans fat: 0 g; Cholesterol: 11.8 mg; Sodium: 582 mg; Total carbohydrates: 43.3 g; Fiber: 3 g; Sugars 6.9 g; Protein: 10.3 g

Grilled Halibut Steak with Pineapple-Lime Salsa

For the salsa

⅓ cup pineapple preserves

¼ cup finely chopped red bell pepper

2 tablespoons finely chopped red onion

1 tablespoon seeded, finely chopped jalapeño pepper

1 teaspoon dried mint flakes *

⅛ teaspoon salt (omit if on a low-sodium diet)

2 tablespoons fresh lime juice

8 ounces canned unsweetened pineapple tidbits, drained

For the fish

1 teaspoon vegetable oil

1 large clove garlic, minced ~

4 4-ounce halibut steaks (about ¾-inch thick)

¼ teaspoon salt (omit if on a low-sodium diet)

Cooking spray

Lime wedges, optional

Cilantro sprigs, optional

To prepare the salsa: Combine all ingredients in a bowl. Stir well. Set aside.

To prepare the fish: In a small bowl, combine oil and garlic; brush over fish. Sprinkle salt over fish; set aside. Heat a grill, broiler, or grill pan; coat with cooking spray. Place fish on grill, and cook for 3 minutes on each side, or until fish flakes easily when tested with a fork.

Spoon the salsa over the fish. Serve with lime wedges, and garnish with cilantro sprigs.

Makes 4 servings

Nutrition information per serving: Calories: 235; Total fat: 3.8 g; Saturated fat: 0.5 g; Trans fat: 0 g; Cholesterol: 35.8 mg; Sodium: 135 mg; Total carbohydrates: 26.2 g; Fiber: 1 g; Sugars: 23.2 g; Protein: 23.8 g

Lentils with Garlic and Rosemary

¾ cup chopped onion
½ cup diced cooked ham
⅓ cup diced carrot
1 teaspoon crushed dried rosemary *
¾ teaspoon dried sage *
¼ teaspoon ground black pepper
⅓ pound dried lentils
4 ounces fat-free beef broth *
2 cloves garlic, chopped ~
1 bay leaf
Chopped fresh parsley, optional

Pour 1½ cups of water into an electric slow cooker (Crock-Pot). Add all ingredients except the parsley. Cook covered on high-heat setting for 3 hours, or until lentils are tender. Remove bay leaf; garnish with parsley before serving.

Makes 4 servings

Nutrition information per serving: Calories: 193; Total fat: 1.8 g; Saturated fat: 0.6 g; Trans fat: 0 g; Cholesterol: 10.3 mg; Sodium: 363 mg; Total carbohydrates: 28.3 g; Fiber: 13.2 g; Sugars: 2.6 g; Protein: 4.8 g

Mixed Mesclun Greens and Apple Salad

For the dressing
¼ cup fresh lemon juice
3 tablespoons honey
1 teaspoon olive oil
Dash of salt
Dash of freshly ground black pepper

For the salad
¼ cup crumbled blue cheese ▪
2 cups chopped (unpeeled) Granny Smith apples
1 cup chopped (unpeeled) Braeburn apples
1 cup chopped (unpeeled) McIntosh apples
2 slices turkey bacon, cooked in a pan or on a panini grill and
    chopped
4 cups mixed salad greens (a packaged mesclun mix works well)

To prepare the dressing: Combine all ingredients in a small bowl; stir well with a whisk.

To prepare the salad: Combine cheese, apples, and bacon in a large bowl. Drizzle the dressing over the apple mixture; toss gently to coat. Divide the greens among four salad plates, and top each with about 1 cup of the apple mixture.

Makes 4 servings

Nutrition information per serving: Calories: 192; Total fat: 6 g; Saturated fat: 2.4 g; Trans fat: 0 g; Cholesterol: 14.2 mg; Sodium: 337 mg; Total carbohydrates: 33 g; Fiber: 3.6 g; Sugars: 26.6 g; Protein: 5.1 g

Slightly Piquant Squash Soup

1¾ cups low-sodium chicken broth *
¾ cup chopped onion
⅛ teaspoon crushed red pepper
1¾ cups cubed acorn squash
⅛ teaspoon salt (omit if on a low-sodium diet)
⅛ cup long-grain rice
2 tablespoons chunky peanut butter
Chopped fresh parsley for garnish

In a large saucepan, bring ¼ cup of the broth to a boil. Add onion and pepper, and cook over high heat until tender, about 5 minutes. Add remaining 1½ cups broth, squash, salt, and 1¾ cups of water. Bring to a boil. Cover, reduce heat, and simmer for 20 minutes. Add rice; cover, and simmer for another 20 minutes, or until squash and rice are tender.

Place peanut butter and half of the soup mixture in a blender or food processor, and process until smooth. Pour the puree into a bowl. Puree the remaining soup, and add to the bowl, stirring well. Return mixture to stove top, and heat for 2 minutes. Divide the soup among four individual bowls. Garnish with parsley.

Makes 4 servings

Nutrition information per serving: Calories: 122; Total fat: 4.8 g; Saturated
    fat: 0.9 g; Trans fat: 0 g; Cholesterol: 0 mg; Sodium: 147 mg; Total
    carbohydrates: 16.8 g; Fiber: 2.2 g; Sugars: 2.1 g; Protein: 5.3 g

Snack Wedges of Sweet Potato with Savory Hummus

For the potato wedges

Cooking spray

2 medium-size sweet potatoes, each cut into 8 wedges

2 tablespoons olive oil

½ teaspoon salt (omit if on a low-sodium diet)

¼ teaspoon garlic powder * ~

½ teaspoon paprika *

¼ teaspoon ground cumin *

For the hummus

2 tablespoons tahini (sesame seed paste)

1½ teaspoons lemon juice

½ teaspoon ground coriander *

½ teaspoon cayenne pepper

5 ounces garbanzo beans, drained

1 clove garlic ~

¼ teaspoon ground cumin *

To prepare the potato wedges: Preheat oven to 450°F. Coat a baking sheet with cooking spray. Place sweet potatoes in a large bowl and drizzle oil over the wedges, tossing well to coat. In a separate bowl, combine salt, garlic powder, paprika, and cumin. Sprinkle over potatoes, and toss well to coat. Arrange the wedges in a single layer on the baking sheet, and bake for 20 minutes, or until tender.

To prepare the hummus: Place all ingredients in a blender or food processor. Process for 4 minutes, or until mixture is smooth. Serve the wedges with the hummus.

Makes 4 servings

Nutrition information per serving: Calories: 202; Total fat: 11.5 g; Saturated fat: 1.6 g; Trans fat: 0 g; Cholesterol: 0 mg; Sodium: 425 mg; Total carbohydrates: 22.2 g; Fiber: 4.4 g; Sugars: 3.9 g; Protein: 4.3 g

Stuffed Clams

8 clams in shells, scrubbed (1 pound)

½ tablespoon cornmeal

½ teaspoon olive oil

¼ cup finely chopped onion

⅓ cup finely chopped shallots

¼ cup finely chopped celery

2 cloves garlic, crushed ~

2 tablespoons finely chopped fresh parsley, plus fresh leaves for
   garnish (optional)

½ teaspoon grated lemon zest

¼ teaspoon dried oregano *

¼ teaspoon dried thyme *

¼ cup fresh bread crumbs, toasted *

¼ teaspoon salt

⅛ teaspoon ground black pepper

Dash of ground red pepper

Place clams in a large bowl, and cover with ½ cup of cold water. Sprinkle with cornmeal, and let stand for 30 minutes. Drain and rinse.

Bring 2 cups of water to a boil in a large Dutch oven. Add the clams, cover, and cook for 4 minutes, or until shells open. Remove the clams from the pan, reserving 1 cup of the cooking liquid. Discard any unopened shells. Allow clams to cool, and then remove meat, chop, and set aside. Reserve eight large shell halves.

Heat oil in a large nonstick skillet over medium-high heat. Add onion, shallots, celery, and garlic; sauté for 3 minutes. Add clam meat, chopped parsley, lemon zest, oregano, and thyme; sauté for 1 minute. Remove from heat. Stir in bread crumbs, salt, black pepper, and red pepper. Add the reserved cooking liquid, stirring until dry ingredients are moistened.

Preheat oven to 350°F. Divide the bread crumb mixture evenly among the eight clam shell halves, pressing mixture gently into shells. Arrange the stuffed shells on a baking sheet, and bake for 20 minutes. Garnish with fresh parsley, and serve hot.

Makes 4 servings (2 stuffed shells per serving)

Nutrition information per serving: Calories: 90.4; Total fat: 1.4 g; Saturated fat: 0.2 g; Trans fat: 0 g; Cholesterol: 12.7 mg; Sodium: 225 mg; Total carbohydrates: 12.6 g; Fiber: 0.9 g; Sugars: 1.1 g; Protein: 6.6 g

Index

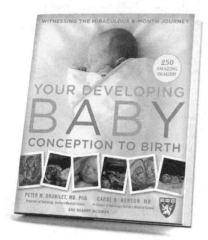
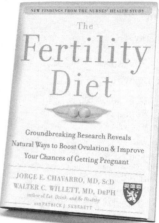
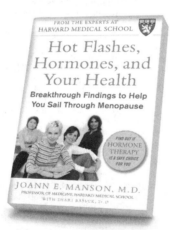
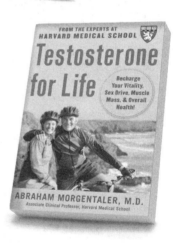
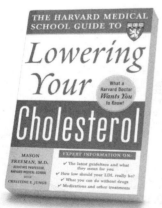
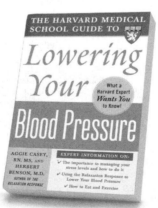